Phil. Trans. R. Soc. Lond. B **325**, 39–44 (1989)   [39]

Printed in Great Britain

EPIDEMIOLOGICAL AND STATISTICAL ASPECTS OF THE AIDS EPIDEMIC: INTRODUCTION

By R. M. ANDERSON, F.R.S.,[1] D. R. COX, F.R.S.,[2] AND HILARY C. HILLIER[3]

[1] *Department of Pure and Applied Biology, Imperial College of Science and Technology, London SW7 2BB, U.K.*
[2] *Nuffield College, Oxford OX1 1NF, U.K.*
[3] *Department of Health, Hannibal House, Elephant and Castle, London SE1 6TE, U.K.*

In 1988, a government working party studied estimates of incidence and prevalence of numbers of acquired immunodeficiency syndrome (AIDS) cases. They investigated a series of epidemiological, statistical and mathematical problems associated with predicting trends in incidences of AIDS.

This paper introduces a series of papers that give a fuller and more technical exposition of the appendixes of that working party report. The papers provide a brief background to the current state of knowledge on the epidemiology of the infection and the disease; a deterministic model for human immunodeficiency virus (HIV) transmission in the male homosexual community in England and Wales is introduced. Back-projection methods are studied in two papers, following the distribution of the incubation period of the disease. The concept of minimum size of the epidemic is introduced. Mathematical functions to describe the spread of HIV infection are refined by using past trends in the incidence of AIDS to estimate values for some parameters.

Survival times for AIDS patients from the point of diagnosis are considered and evidence for changes in male homosexual sexual behaviour is studied; lag-time from the point of diagnosis to the report of the case is also examined. There is a comparative analysis of the AIDS epidemic in various European countries. The incubation period of HIV in patients with haemophilia A and B infections and the problems associated with making predictions for different at-risk groups or small sub-groups based on geographical area are discussed.

Reasons for fluctuation between the number of reported cases from month to month are provided.

In March 1988 a small working party was established by the Chief Medical Officers of England and Wales. The working party reported 'on predictions, for a 2–5 year period, in England and Wales, of incidence and prevalence estimates for numbers of live cases of acquired immunodeficiency syndrome (AIDS) and, where adequate information is available, of other human immunodeficiency virus (HIV)-associated conditions, on the number of deaths and on the overall numbers of HIV-infected individuals; and considered the means for updating such predictions, and to make recommendations'. (HMSO 1988).

The members of the working party were: Sir David Cox (Chairman); Professor R. M. Anderson; Dr Anne M. Johnson, Senior Lecturer in Epidemiology, Academic Department of Genito–Urinary Medicine, University College and Middlesex School of Medicine; Professor M. J. R. Healy, London School of Hygiene and Tropical Medicine; Dr Valerie Isham, Department of Statistical Science, University College London; Professor A. D. Wilkie, Consulting Actuary, Messrs R. Watson and Sons; Dr N. E. Day, Director, MRC Biostatistics

Unit, Cambridge; Dr O. N. Gill, Consultant Epidemiologist, PHLS Communicable Disease Surveillance Centre; Dr Anna McCormick, Consultant Epidemiologist, PHLS Communicable Disease Surveillance Centre; Secretariat: Dr Gillian Greenberg, Senior Medical Officer, Department of Health; Mrs Hilary Hillier.

The members of the working party investigated a series of epidemiological, statistical and mathematical problems associated with making predictions of future trends in the incidences of AIDS and infection with the etiological agent of the disease, the human immunodeficiency virus type 1 (HIV-1). The final report, which was published in November 1988, contained a series of appendixes giving brief details of parts of the research that underpinned the major conclusions in the main body of the text. We felt that the work outlined in these appendixes required fuller and more technical exposition so that public health workers, epidemiologists, medical and scientific researchers in the U.K. and other countries could assess in more detail the methods, assumptions and associated problems that surround the issue of making predictions about future trends in the incidences of AIDS and HIV infection.

This issue contains eleven papers that describe various aspects of the research, ranging from studies of the transmission dynamics of HIV, via epidemiological work on temporal changes in patterns of sexual behaviour, to statistical studies of the relation between AIDS incidence and the number of people infected with HIV, and the survival-time distribution of AIDS patients. The research reported in these papers was completed over the 5–6 month lifespan of the working party and hence much of it is preliminary in character and highlights problems as opposed to solutions. However, we feel the field is of sufficient practical and scientific importance to merit the publication of these contributions within a single issue.

The problems that surround making predictions about future trends in AIDS incidence are somewhat daunting. Indeed, if practical consideration did not demand the provision of such information (however tentative in character) for health care planning, scientific judgement alone would argue for extreme caution in the production and interpretation of projections. The reasons for this are at least threefold. First, the disease and its etiological agent have only recently been diagnosed (AIDS was first characterized in 1981 and the virus HIV-1 isolated in 1983). Although progress in understanding the basic biology of the virus, in particular the structure and function of its genome, has been rapid, much remains uncertain about key processes that determine transmission within communities of people. Epidemiological data have accumulated slowly, largely because of the very long (and highly variable) incubation period (the period from first infection to the diagnosis of the disease AIDS). Current estimates based on transfusion associated cases and infections in injecting drug users (IDUS) and male homosexuals suggest a median period of 8–10 years. The implication of this is that epidemiological data will only accumulate slowly over decades of longitudinal study of infected persons and cohorts. In addition, one of the primary routes of transmission is via sexual contact. This poses additional problems for epidemiological study, given the sensitivities of individuals, societies and government bodies to open discussion and investigation of the behavioural characteristics that influence transmission via this pathway. Epidemiological uncertainties therefore limit the accuracy of projections based on mathematical models of transmission within populations, even within a particular at risk group (e.g. male homosexuals), let alone between and within the different groups that are at risk from infection and disease.

The second reason concerns the quality of the epidemiological data upon which projections into the future are based. In England and Wales we benefit from a good infectious disease

Phil. Trans. R. Soc. Lond. B **325**, 37–187 (1989)   [37]

Printed in Great Britain

EPIDEMIOLOGICAL AND STATISTICAL ASPECTS OF THE AIDS EPIDEMIC

(Compiled and edited by D. R. Cox, F.R.S., R. M. Anderson, F.R.S., and Hilary C. Hillier –
Typescripts received **20** *March* **1989**)

CONTENTS

reporting system, based at the Public Health Laboratory Service Communicable Disease Surveillance Centre at Colindale. However, the very nature of the disease and its temporal relation with the point of first infection, implies that current reports of the incidence of the disease AIDS represent infection events that happened, on average, several years ago. They therefore represent only a small fraction of the total number of people currently infected with HIV. Data on the prevalence of infection in different risk groups, and in the general population, are very limited at present. Good data on both the incidence of disease and infection would greatly enhance our ability to project into the future. One of the major recommendations of our report, therefore, was to instigate, as a matter of urgency, studies to improve understanding of the number of people currently infected with the virus. Shortly before the publication of the report, the U.K. Government announced that it saw neither legal obstacle nor ethical objection to anonymous screening. The Medical Research Council has been invited to submit proposals for studies based on anonymous and named testing. Although these steps fall short of a large scale random survey of the general population, they represent a significant step towards improving the quality of the epidemiological data base, taking account of the many practical and ethical problems that surround screening for HIV infection. Linked to the need for data on the prevalence of HIV infection as well as the incidence of AIDS, is the need for large scale, longitudinal studies of sexual behaviour both in particular risk groups and the general population. Even with good data on HIV prevalence in samples of individuals drawn from particular risk groups, projection requires knowledge of the size of the at risk population. One of the appendixes to the report discussed the problems of estimating the numbers of persons infected with HIV from the information currently available and concluded that the uncertainties involved were considerable. Information on the size of the risk groups, especially those most at risk, homosexuals and IVDUS, is scant, and the existing studies on seroprevalence in these populations are likely to be biased because all rely to a greater or lesser extent on self-selected samples. Applying the available information, the report concluded that the number infected by the end of 1987 was probably between 20000 and 50000, though it could plausibly lie outside this range. Our ignorance of the numbers of those within each risk group, without which more precise estimates cannot be made, can only be abated by large scale detailed studies of behaviour. The implementation of such research was a further recommendation of the report.

The third problem area is intimately linked with the other areas. It concerns the influence of education and publicity on patterns of behaviour, and hence infection with HIV, during the course of the epidemic in the U.K. A brief comparison of epidemiological trends in the United States of America and the U.K. suggests that the virus began to spread somewhat later in male homosexual and drug injecting communities in Europe than in those in North America. The knowledge of what was happening in the U.S.A., linked with the extensive publicity and education campaign mounted by the government in the U.K. in 1986, appear to have resulted in significant changes of behaviour amongst certain at risk groups, particularly male homosexuals, in England and Wales around 1984–85. These changes are thought to have had an impact on the rate of spread of the virus, but we are ignorant, in quantitative terms, of the temporal pattern of change in either the incidence of new HIV infection or sexual behaviour. Given our ignorance of many key epidemiological parameters, making projections is difficult enough in the absence of secular temporal trends. The problem is made much more difficult by unknown temporal changes in certain key parameters.

[3]

In the face of such uncertainty it is essential to try to synthesize conclusions from a variety of approaches to making predictions about future trends. This is apparent in the papers in this issue. It is organized as follows. The first paper by Anderson *et al.* provides a brief background to the current state of knowledge on the epidemiology of the infection and the disease. The paper then addresses the problem of formulating a deterministic mathematical model of HIV transmission in the male homosexual community of England and Wales, which incorporates distributed incubation and infectious periods plus heterogeneity in sexual activity. Parameter estimates are, where possible, based on empirical information and sensitivity analyses are performed to assess the significance of variation in parameter assignments and changes in sexual behaviour. This paper is followed by one by Wilkie in which a similar approach is adopted using actuarial models to follow the history of cohorts of people. It has the added refinement of age structure, but the simplification of homogeneity in sexual behaviour.

The next two papers, by Isham and Day & Gore, adopt a different approach, based on back projection of the number infected with HIV on the basis of current data on the incidence of AIDS. This approach, which uses convolution methods, requires information (or assumptions) on the distribution of the incubation period of the disease (e.g. Weibull or gamma in form). Projections can be made into the future provided a further set of assumptions is made concerning the incidence of new HIV infections over the period of the projections. The 'minimum size' of the epidemic can be estimated if one assumes that all transmission ceases at the present time point and that projections of future cases of AIDS are based on current and past history of the number infected with the virus. The fifth paper by Cox & Medley adopts a further approach that is arguably the most practically useful with respect to making short term projections over one to a few years ahead. It relies on the choice of a mathematical function (perhaps based on studies of simple mathematical models of epidemic processes) and the estimation of its parameters from past trends in the incidence of AIDS. Taking account of the distributed (and time varying) delay between diagnosis and report, these estimates can be used to make projections into the future. The linear–logistic function appears at present to provide a reasonable description of past events. Interestingly, simple mathematical models of HIV transmission incorporating distributed incubation and infectious periods or heterogeneity (or both) in sexual activity generate an epidemic curve that is well described by the linear–logistic model.

The remaining papers address specific epidemiological or statistical issues: Reeves considers the survival times of AIDS patients from the point of diagnosis, and formulates a simple model for the distribution. Johnson & Gill weigh the evidence for behavioural changes in different at risk groups over the past ten years, thereby addressing one of the key problems surrounding projection. McCormick examines age stratified reports of mortality among males and females in England and Wales during the period of the AIDS epidemic to assess whether or not there is any evidence for under-reporting of AIDS associated mortality. A comparative study of the rate of growth of the AIDS epidemic in various European countries is provided by Mariotto. Darby & Doll examine the distribution of the incubation period in patients with haemophilia A and B via longitudinal studies. Finally, Cox & Davison examine the problem of making projections for different at risk groups or for small sub-groups based on geographical areas.

It is important to stress the preliminary nature of many of the reported studies, and the great uncertainties involved in making projections. The original report was written in the summer of 1988, and was based on cases of AIDS and HIV infection reported up to June 1988. We now have the benefit of a further 9 months' data and it is interesting to see whether this alters the general conclusions of the report. The number of cases of AIDS reported by June 1988 had already shown some signs that the early exponential growth had given way to a phase of much slower and more linear growth (table 1). Although there is considerable fluctuation in the numbers of reported cases from month to month, and even from quarter to quarter, it is now apparent that the number of reports each quarter increased relatively slowly between the middle of 1987 and the end of 1988. A similar pattern has occurred in other countries, notably the F.R.G., France and Australia.

TABLE 1. MONTH OF REPORTED AIDS CASES IN ENGLAND AND WALES

month	1982	1983	1984	1985	year 1986	1987	1988	1989
January	—	1	5	11	12	57	51	64
February	—	1	2	12	15	51	57	52
March	2	0	5	11	21	26	78	83
April	—	0	2	17	6	19	28	—
May	—	5	4	5	24	40	76	—
June	—	1	3	10	25	73	49	—
July	—	2	5	19	59	53	68	—
August	—	2	9	8	20	68	59	—
September	—	6	11	14	16	54	62	—
October	—	3	10	16	49	49	67	—
November	—	1	8	14	21	45	61	—
December	—	4	9	14	22	53	51	—
total	2	26	73	151	290	588	707	199

There are several possible explanations for this. In their paper, Anderson *et al.* suggest that a slowing down in the rate of growth of new cases is consistent with a model of the epidemic in male homosexuals in which the average number of sexual partners is assumed to be sharply reduced after 1985. This model would predict an epidemic that peaks in 1989–1990, and is consistent with between 10000 and 15000 homosexuals being infected at the period of peak incidence; this is at the bottom end of the probable range of values suggested by applying estimates of seroprevalence to estimates of the size of the homosexual population. Under this, relatively optimistic assumption, the peak of the epidemic for homosexuals has almost been reached, though the number of cases might still go on rising slowly for some time after 1990 because of cases arising in the heterosexual and drug-using communities.

A further possibility is that the flattening in the number of reported cases is an artefact, caused by what the Americans have called 'reporting fatigue', i.e. an increasing tendency to late reporting or to not reporting at all. However, there is no evidence that reporting lags are lengthening and the fact that a similar phenomenon has occurred in other countries, with identical timing and to a very similar degree, makes this seem an unlikely explanation.

A third possible situation is that treatment with the drug zidovudine (AZT) may prolong the incubation period for those to whom it is administered before the onset of AIDS, in addition to prolonging survival time among those with AIDS. Zidovudine started to be used quite widely in this country around the end of 1986. The effect would be a once and for all lengthening of the average incubation period for those given zidovudine, though by how much is very uncertain, causing a lateral shift in the incidence curve. If this is the explanation, then the numbers of cases will start to rise again more rapidly once this effect has worked through. This theory would explain the similar flattening in reports of new cases in other countries. It is worth noting that in France the most recent figures show a return to faster growth towards the end of 1988 (although the epidemic there has rather different characteristics from that in this country and the numbers of new cases were rising faster in France than in England and Wales before the levelling off occurred in both countries in 1987).

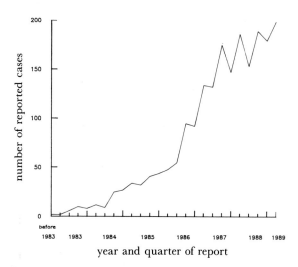

FIGURE 1. New cases of AIDS reported to the Communicable Disease Surveillance Centre by March 1989 for England and Wales.

All these uncertainties highlight the need to: (*a*) continuously update projections as data and biological understanding improve; (*b*) develop better methods for projection, perhaps based on seeking simple mathematical functions that approximate the patterns generated by complex transmission models; (*c*) refine techniques for parameter estimation taking account of the variability that seems to pervade the pattern of HIV infection and disease, both at the individual and population levels and, most importantly; (*d*) encourage the acquisition of better and more extensive epidemiological and behavioural data via nationally coordinated research programmes.

Phil. Trans. R. Soc. Lond. B **325**, 45–98 (1989)   [45]

Printed in Great Britain

THE TRANSMISSION DYNAMICS OF THE HUMAN IMMUNODEFICIENCY VIRUS TYPE 1 IN THE MALE HOMOSEXUAL COMMUNITY IN THE UNITED KINGDOM: THE INFLUENCE OF CHANGES IN SEXUAL BEHAVIOUR

By R. M. ANDERSON,[1] F.R.S., S. P. BLYTHE,[2] S. GUPTA[1] and E. KONINGS[1]

[1] *Department of Pure and Applied Biology, Imperial College of Science and Technology, London SW7 2BB, U.K.*

[2] *Physics Department, Strathclyde University, John Anderson Building,* 107 *Rottenrow, Glasgow G4 0NG, U.K.*

This paper examines the transmission dynamics of human immune deficiency virus type 1 (HIV-1) in the male homosexual population in the U.K. via numerical studies employing a mathematical model representing the principal epidemiological process. The model is based on an assumption of proportionate mixing between different sexual-activity classes (defined by the rate of sexual partner change per unit of time) and incorporates heterogeneity in sexual activity, distributed infection and incubation periods and the recruitment of susceptibles to the sexually active population. The sensitivity of model predictions to various assumptions and parameter assignments is examined. Numerical studies of model behaviour focus on the influence of changes in the magnitudes of the transmission parameters, associated with three periods of infectiousness during the incubation period of acquired immune deficiency syndrome (AIDS), on the magnitude and duration of the epidemic and on the level of the endemic equilibrium state. Predicted temporal trends in the incidence of AIDS are shown to be particularly sensitive to changes in the intensities and durations of the stages of infectiousness. Most of the paper addresses the influence of changes in sexual behaviour on the magnitude and duration of the epidemic. Numerical simulations show that the manner in which behavioural changes occur and who is influenced by such changes (i.e. infecteds or susceptibles, the sexually active population or new recruits to this population) have a major impact on the future timecourse of the epidemic. The greatest reduction in the incidence of AIDS over the coming decades is induced by changes in the rate of sexual-partner change among the sexually active population, particularly those currently infected. The time periods at which changes in behaviour occur, in relation to the starting point of the epidemic (assumed to be 1979), are also of particular significance to the future pattern of the incidence of disease and infection. Changes in behaviour early on in the timecourse of the epidemic have a much greater impact than equivalent changes at latter time points. On the basis of limited data on the pattern of change in sexual behaviour among the male homosexual community in the U.K., numerical studies of model behaviour tentatively suggest that the epidemic is at, or near to, a period of peak incidence of the disease AIDS. Analyses suggest that, following the peak in incidence, there will be a period of slow decline over many decades provided recent changes in behaviour are maintained in the coming years. The difficulties surrounding model formulation and the prediction of future trends are stressed. Many uncertainties remain concerning parameter assignments and emphasis is placed on the need for better data on patterns of sexual behaviour and changes therein, infectiousness throughout the long and variable incubation period of AIDS and the number of individuals currently infected with HIV-1 in the U.K.

1. Introduction

Mathematical models of infection and disease may serve as illuminating caricatures of observed pattern and current hypotheses, as analytic tools for the estimation of epidemiological parameters, as guides to the information needed to improve understanding and as a template for planning health-care provision and programmes of control. Over the past few years increasing attention has been focused on the application of statistical and mathematical methods to the study of the epidemiology of the acquired immune deficiency syndrome (AIDS) and the transmission dynamics of the aetiological agent of the disease, the human immunodeficiency virus type 1 (HIV-1) (Anderson 1988 a).

This research falls into five broad areas. The first concerns short-term prediction of the number of cases of AIDS by the use of simple mathematical functions such as the exponential or the logistic (Norman 1985; McEvoy & Tillet 1985). The parameters of the models may be estimated by fitting the functions to the recorded longitudinal patterns of AIDS incidence, and various refinements may be included such as a distributed lag between diagnosis and reporting (Cox & Medley 1989). The second area is the use of models to estimate particular epidemiological parameters such as the rate of infection per head, the probability of transmission per sexual contact and summary statistics of the distribution of the incubation period (Lui et al. 1986; Medley et al. 1987; Grant & Wiley 1987; Winkelstein et al. 1987; May & Anderson 1987; Anderson 1988 b). The fourth area is the development of models to describe the dynamic interaction between HIV-1 and the human immune system within individual patients. To date this area has received little attention but it is an important topic for future research (Cooper 1986; Anderson 1988 a). The fifth and final area is the subject of this paper and concerns the development of models to describe the transmission dynamics of the virus within and between defined at-risk groups. Most past studies have centred on the principal at-risk group, namely, male homosexuals, in developed countries (Anderson et al. 1986; Dietz & Hadeler 1988; Hymen & Stanley 1988; May & Anderson 1988). This group currently accounts for more than 70% of reported cases in countries such as the U.S.A. and the U.K.

In this paper we examine the transmission dynamics of HIV-1 in the male homosexual population in the U.K. via the development and analysis of a simple model that incorporates distributed infectious and incubation periods, heterogeneity in sexual activity (defined as the number of different sexual partners per unit of time) and continual recruitment of susceptible individuals to the population. The model is based on published research (see Anderson et al. 1986, 1987; Anderson & May 1986; May & Anderson 1987; Blythe & Anderson 1988 a, b, c) and the paper examines the sensitivity of model predictions to various assumptions and parameter assignments via extensive numerical studies. The primary focus of these analyses is an assessment of the influence of changes in sexual behaviour on the likely course of the epidemic in the coming decades.

The paper is organized as follows. The first section provides a very brief overview of recent progress towards an understanding of the major epidemiological processes that determine the pattern of the epidemic in the male homosexual community. The second section outlines the structure of the model and the various assumptions made in its formulation. Particular attention is given to the formulation of the transmission term and the treatment of distributed infectious and incubation periods. The third and longest section summarizes the results of extensive numerical investigations of the properties of the model by reference to temporal trends in the incidence of disease (AIDS) and the proportion of the community infected (seroprevalence) with HIV-1, stratified by sexual activity class (the rate of change in sexual partners). The final discussion section pays particular attention given to the influence of changes in sexual behaviour on the likely pattern of the epidemic in the U.K. over the coming decades.

2. EPIDEMIOLOGICAL PATTERNS AND PARAMETERS

The overall pattern of spread of HIV infection within a defined risk group depends on the magnitude of the basic reproductive rate, R_0, which measures the number of new cases of infection produced, on average, by an infected individual in the early stages of the epidemic when virtually all contacts are susceptible. The basic reproductive rate is a composite parameter formed from the product of the average probability β, that an infected individual will infect a susceptible sexual partner over the duration of their relationship, multiplied by the effective average number of new partners acquired per unit of time, c (within the specified risk-group), multiplied by the average duration of infectiousness, D:

$$R_0 = \beta c D. \tag{1}$$

There are, of course many problems associated with what exactly is meant by 'average' with respect to the three components in this definition. These problems are addressed in the following section on model formulation. The quantity R_0 simply helps to focus attention on what must be measured to gain a crude understanding of the pattern of spread of infection (Anderson *et al.* 1986; May & Anderson 1987, 1988).

Since the discovery of the aetiological agents of AIDS, much research has been directed towards the measurement of the components encapsulated in the definition of R_0. However, many uncertainties remain, largely as a result of the long and variable incubation period of the disease (many years) and as a consequence of public and professional sensitivities surrounding the study of sexual behaviour in human communities. A recent review of progress towards parameter assignments that indicates the problems and uncertainties that are emerging in such research is given by Anderson & May (1988). In this section we briefly summarize current understanding and indicate the major areas of uncertainty.

(a) *The proportion of infecteds who develop AIDS*

Prospective studies of homosexual men infected with HIV show that the rate of progression from infection to AIDS is slow. The rate of progression appears to vary with time from infection, being low in the first year and rising thereafter. Estimates of the fraction f who will go on to develop AIDS have increased with time. Rates of progression from seropositivity to AIDS derived from cohorts where the dates of seroconversion are not always known range from less than 1 % to more than 12 % per year with an average around 5–7 %. Rates of progression to AIDS are much higher in perinatally infected young children as well as in elderly people, by comparison with sexually active adults. Current evidence suggests that between 30 and 75 % of infected individuals will have progressed to AIDS within six years. Overall, it is likely that a very high fraction (perhaps greater than 90 %) will ultimately progress to AIDS with the only uncertainty being the distribution of times to the development of disease (table 1). Therapy with azidothymidine is likely to influence this distribution because studies suggest that the drug

TABLE 1. PROPORTION (p) OF HIV ANTIBODY POSITIVE INDIVIDUALS DEVELOPING AIDS

risk group	sample size	observation time (months)	p	reference
haemophiliacs	18	24	0.06	Simmonds et al. (1988)
haemophiliacs	40	36	0.13	Goedert et al. (1986)
haemophiliacs	92	48	0.11	Eyster et al. (1987)
haemophiliacs	84	54	0.12	Eyster et al. (1987)
haemophiliacs	77	?	0.13	Jason et al. (1988)
iv drug users	165	9	0.02	Des Jarlais et al. (1987)
iv drug users	72	14	0.06	Vaccher et al. (1988)
iv drug users	77	18	0.07	Zulaica et al. (1988)
iv drug users	50	24	0.32	Fernandez-Cruz et al. (1988)
iv drug users	181	24	0.12	Selwyn et al. (1988)
iv drug users	102	36	0.09	Crovari et al. (1988)
iv drug users	24	36	0.13	Goedert et al. (1986)
ex-iv drug users	61	36	0.03	Crovari et al. (1988)
PGL patients	88	15	0.08	Weller et al. (1985)
PGL patients	90	19	0.17	Weller et al. (1985)
PGL patients	101	20	0.60	Gottlieb et al. (1987)
PGL patients	100	24	0.13	Carne et al. (1987)
PGL patients	22	35	0.46	Harrer et al. (1988)
PGL patients	42	60	0.29	Weller et al. (1985)
PGL patients	200	61	0.08	Abrams et al. (1985)
PGL patients	200	74	0.38	Abrams et al. (1988)
PGL patients	75	72	0.38	Kaplan et al. (1988)
PGL & ARC patients	68	20	0.76	Gottlieb et al. (1987)
homosexuals	1835	15	0.03	Polk et al. (1987)
homosexuals	813	18	0.07	Gottlieb et al. (1987)
homosexuals	233	24	0.80	Antonen et al. (1987)
homosexuals	42	24	0.14	Detels et al. (1987)
homosexuals	306	30	0.10	de Wolf et al. (1988)
homosexuals	30	31	0.23	Gerstoft et al. (1987)
homosexuals	96	32.5	0.70	Schechter et al. (1988)
homosexuals	34	36	0.26	Pederson et al. (1987)
homosexuals	33	36	0.12	Weber et al. (1986)
homosexuals	86	36	0.22	Goedert et al. (1987)
homosexuals	44	36	0.34	Goedert et al. (1986)
homosexuals	288	44	0.17	Moss et al. (1988)
homosexuals	42	36	0.17	Goedert et al. (1986)
homosexuals	26	36	0.08	Goedert et al. (1986)
homosexuals	18	48	0.22	El-Sadr et al. (1987)
homosexuals	30	48	0.07	Titti et al. (1988)
homosexuals	246	50	0.15	Schechter et al. (1988)
homosexuals	115	53	0.28	Karlsson et al. (1988)
homosexuals	86	60	0.56	Biggar et al. (1988)
homosexuals	31	61	0.06	Jaffe (1985)
homosexuals	1100	72	0.04	Curran et al. (1985)
homosexuals	71	86	0.42	Hessol et al. (1988)
mothers	16	30	0.31	Scott et al. (1985)
children of HIV + mothers	178	12	0.60	European Collaborative Study (1988)

suppresses viral replication in certain patients (Parks et al. 1988). Whether or not drug treatment will prevent the development of AIDS in some patients over very long time periods (i.e. decades) is uncertain at present.

(b) *The incubation period of AIDS*

A variety of parametric and non-parametric methods have been used to estimate summary statistics of the incubation periods of AIDS (defined as the time interval between infection and the diagnosis of symptoms of disease) (see Lui *et al.* 1986; Medley *et al.* 1987, 1988). A summary of published estimates of certain statistics (e.g. the mean or the median) is presented in table 2 for various risk groups.

TABLE 2. INCUBATION PERIOD

risk group	incubation/years mean	median	sample size	reference
U.S.A. heterosexual prisoners, IV drug abusers	1.91	—	14	Hanrahan *et al.* (1984)
U.S.A. homosexuals	0.88	—	12	Auerbach *et al.* (1984)
U.S.A. TA adults over 13 years	4.5	—	83	Lui *et al.* (1986)
U.S.A. TA adults	15	—	144	Rees (1987)
U.K. TA cases	3.1	—	393	MRC/DHSS project (1987)
U.S.A. TA adults 60 years+	5.5	5.44	135	Medley *et al.* (1987)
U.S.A. TA persons below 5 and 59 years	8.23	7.97	126	Medley *et al.* (1987)
U.S.A. TA female cases	8.7	8.36	112	Medley *et al.* (1987)
U.S.A. TA male cases	5.62	5.5	185	Medley *et al.* (1987)
U.S.A. TA children under 12 years	1.97	1.9	36	Medley *et al.* (1987)
U.S.A. TA children under 12 years	2.03	—	40	Rogers *et al.* (1987)
U.S.A. TA children under 12 years	2.58	—	90	Rogers *et al.* (1988)
U.S.A. perinatally infected under 12 years	—	5.4	215	Auger *et al.* (1988)
U.S.A. children	—	0.5 to 5.5	190	Lawrence *et al.* (1988)
U.S.A. TA cases	7.29	7.63	440	Valleron *et al.* (1988)
U.S.A. TA cases				
(Weibull)	4.93	5.21	—	Valleron *et al.* (1988)
(Gamma)	14.11	11.38	—	Valleron *et al.* (1988)
U.S.A. TA adults over 12 years				
(Weibull)	7.59	7.32	512	Medley *et al.* (1988)
(Gamma)	24.07	20.84	—	Medley *et al.* (1988)
U.S.A. Haemophiliacs over 12 years				
(Weibull)	7.66	7.43	1401	Anderson, Medley (1988)
(Gamma)	14.33	12.61	—	Anderson, Medley (1988)

Parametric approaches to the estimation of the distribution of incubation periods in cohorts of individuals within a given risk group (i.e. male homosexuals, intravenous drug users, perinatally infected infants and haemophiliacs), for whom times of infection or seroconversion are known, are based on the development of simple mathematical models. These must take into account the growth in the number of infected individuals through time (i.e. exponential in the early stages of the epidemic), the proportion of infecteds who will ultimately develop AIDS and the form of the probability distribution of the incubation period. With respect to the last, the Weibull and γ-distributions have been used in many of the published studies (see Lui *et al.* 1986; Medley *et al.* 1987, 1988). In the context of the construction of models of the transmission dynamics of the virus, a parametric assumption concerning the form of the distribution is essential for predicting future patterns or trends. Published estimates of the means of Weibull and γ-distributions fitted to observed data (where only a given fraction of the distribution has been observed to date) have wide confidence limits (Kalbfleisch & Lawless 1988). However, for transfusion-associated cases and cases in male homosexuals as well as in intravenous (IV) drug users, estimates of the mean tend to lie in the range of 6–8 years (see table 2). This average appears to be somewhat less in children (less than 12 years) and elderly people (greater than 60 years). The disease in infants infected perinatally appears to have a very short incubation period with averages in the range of 1–3 years (Rogers *et al.* 1987).

(c) *Infectious period*

The average period during which infected individuals are infectious to susceptible partners, over the long and variable incubation period of AIDS, is difficult to measure. Clinical data are accumulating on fluctuations in antigenaemia in infected patients throughout the incubation period (Pederson *et al.* 1987) and one hypothesis is that the peaks in antigenaemia correlate with peaks in infectiousness (Albert *et al.* 1988). As yet, data to support this hypothesis are limited (see Laurian *et al.* 1989) and a growing body of evidence points to wide variation in the likelihood that the virus is transmitted during a single sexual encounter. One approach to the study of infectiousness is to monitor the sexual partners of infected individuals to ascertain the likelihood of transmission to a susceptible partner at various time periods after seroconversion of the initially infected partner. Few such studies have been undertaken so far (table 3). In some cases the virus was transmitted after a single or few sexual contacts whereas in other cases no transmission occurred despite a high frequency of contact (Peterman *et al.* 1987).

Longitudinal studies of fluctuation in HIV antigen concentration in serum from infected patients provide some clues to what might generate such variability. Analyses of the available data on temporal fluctuation in antigen concentrations (assumed to reflect, in some manner, viral abundance and possibly infectiousness) reveal low concentrations (if at all detectable) before seroconversion (about 30–40 days), high concentrations during primary HIV infection (which has an average incubation period of around 40 days) which remain high for a few months before falling to low levels during the asymptomatic phase of the infection. As patients progress to persistent generalized lymphadenopathy (PGL) and AIDS-related complex (ARC) and finally to AIDS, antigen concentration (particularly the p24 core antigen) rises again to high levels.

This pattern suggests tentatively that there are two periods of peak infectiousness (assuming that antigen concentration reflects infectiousness), one shortly after infection lasting for a few months, and one as patients progress to ARC and AIDS, perhaps lasting for a few years (Pedersen *et al.* 1987; Anderson 1988*a*; Anderson & May 1988). It is important to remember, however, that the incubation period of AIDS is very variable between infected individuals and in some people antigen remains detectable and often at high levels of concentration throughout the course of infection. In these patients disease appears to progress rapidly (Moss 1988; Allain *et al.* 1987; Goudsmit *et al.* 1986). The hypothesis of two periods of peak infectiousness remains tentative at present.

The most striking feature of clinical data on antigen fluctuation, and of epidemiological data on the likelihood of transmission, is the high degree of variability between patients or sexual partners (Anderson & Medley 1988).

(d) *Transmission probability*

For the purpose of the models discussed in this paper we define the transmission probability, β, as the average probability that an infected individual will infect a susceptible partner over the duration of their relationship (i.e. defined per partner as opposed to per sexual contact). The form of this definition is in part determined by the character of the epidemiological data used to derive crude estimates of the likelihood of transmission, and in part by the structure of the simple mathematical models employed to study transmission (see Anderson *et al.* 1986; May & Anderson 1988). Data on the magnitude of β is limited at present and that which has

[12]

TABLE 3. PROBABILITY OF HETEROSEXUAL TRANSMISSION, p

(n = sample size)

risk group of index case	p	n	reference
	male to female		
transfusion	0.16	50	Peterman et al. (1988)
transfusion	0.18	55	Peterman & Curran (1986)
mixed including bisexuals	0.07	217	Garcia et al. (1988)
mixed including bisexuals	0.23	97	Padian et al. (1987)
mixed including bisexuals	0.24	132	Padian et al. (1988)
mixed including bisexuals	0.24	41	Johnson et al. (1988)
mixed including bisexuals	0.28	104	De Vincenzi et al. (1988)
mixed including bisexuals	0.28	18	Roumelioutou-Karayannis et al. (1988)
mixed including bisexuals	0.40	68	Stasewski et al. (1988)
mixed including bisexuals	0.45	114	Steigbigel et al. (1988)
mixed including bisexuals	0.50	28	Fischl et al. (1988)
mixed including bisexuals	0.55	75	Sion et al. (1988)
African connections	0.53	62	Laga et al. (1988)
patients from Africa	0.61	150	Hira et al. (1988)
patients from Africa	0.71	14	Sewankambo et al. (1987)
patients from Africa	0.73	38	Taelman et al. (1987)
army personnel	0.33	18	Anderson & May (1988)
iv drug users	0.17	60	Johnson et al. (1988)
iv drug users	0.33	6	Roumelioutou-Karayannis et al. (1988)
iv drug users	0.35	48	Anderson & May (1988)
iv drug users	0.38	71	Milazzo et al. (1988)
iv drug users	0.48	88	Anderson & May (1988)
haemophiliac	0.00	36	Brettler et al. (1988)
haemophiliac	0.03	30	Miller et al. (1987)
haemophiliac	0.04	77	Jones et al. (1985)
haemophiliac	0.04	25	Roumelioutou-Karayannis et al. (1988)
haemophiliac	0.05	21	Lawrence et al. (1988)
haemophiliac	0.06	33	Jason et al. (1986)
haemophiliac	0.07	148	Allain et al. (1986)
haemophiliac	0.10	164	Kamradt et al. (1988)
haemophiliac	0.10	21	Kreiss et al. (1985)
haemophiliac	0.10	40	Biberfeld et al. (1986)
haemophiliac	0.11	35	Lawrence et al. (1988)
haemophiliac	0.13	124	Goedert et al. (1988)
haemophiliac	0.17	21	Winkelstein et al. (1986)
haemophiliac	0.17	24	Goedert et al. (1987)
	female to male		
transfusion	0.08	25	Peterman et al. (1988)
army personnel	0.33	6	Anderson & May (1988)
African connections	0.13	16	Laga et al. (1988)
patients from Africa	0.40	10	Taelman et al. (1987)
patients from Africa	0.73	78	Hira et al. (1988)
iv drug users	0.08	13	Johnson et al. (1988)
iv drug users	0.58	12	Steigbigel et al. (1987)
mixed	0.00	20	Padian et al. (1987)
mixed	0.04	27	De Vincenzi et al. (1988)
mixed	0.09	30	Stasewski et al. (1988)
mixed	0.50	14	Steigbigel et al. (1988)
mixed	0.71	17	Fischl et al. (1987)

been published is characterized by a high degree of variability between studies (table 3). Estimates range from less than 10 % to over 60 %. This variability probably reflects factors such as difference in the frequency and type of sexual contact between partnerships, and in the timing of contact during the long incubation period of the disease in the index case.

As defined above, β is an average value for the likelihood of transmission over the duration of the incubation period of AIDS. If there are two peak periods of infectious, one early and one late in the progression of the disease, it may be better to consider three separate values of β (i.e. β_i) for the first peak in infectiousness, the asymptomatic phase and the late peak of infectiousness, respectively. An additional variable is the average time, T_i, spent in each of these three phases of disease progression.

(e) Sexual activity

The frequency distribution of the rate at which an individual acquires new sexual partners per unit of time (e.g. one year) is an important determinant of the pattern and rate of spread of HIV in a defined community. Simple models of the transmission dynamics of HIV, based on the assumption of proportional mixing (see Hethcote & Yorke 1984; Anderson et al. 1986) suggest that the effective rate of partner change, c, should be defined as the mean of the distribution, m, plus the variance to mean ratio, σ^2/m (May & Anderson 1987):

$$c = m + \sigma^2/m. \tag{2}$$

This definition makes clear the importance of an understanding of the full distribution of the rate of sexual partner change in any analysis of the course of the epidemic. Various studies, based on interviews and the completion of confidential questionnaires, have attempted to define this distribution in samples drawn at various time points, from various male homosexual communities (Fay et al. 1989). Sampling procedures have ranged from quota to random methodologies (see Anderson (1988b) and Anderson & Johnson (1989) for recent reviews of published studies). Survey design and sampling methods for the collection of data on rates of sexual partner change present many problems (Cohen 1987). The studies in the U.K. that have been published so far reveal great variability both in type of sexual activity and in partner change rate, with dependencies on variables such as age, social status and the geographical location from which the sample was drawn (McKusick et al. 1985; Carne et al. 1985; British Market Research Board (BMRB) 1987).

An interesting feature of the data is the existence of a general relation between the mean (m) and variance (σ^2) of the recorded distributions of sexual partner change of power law from:

$$\sigma^2 = am^b. \tag{3}$$

The coefficients a and b can be estimated by regression techniques from a logarithmic plot of σ^2 against m for all published values of the two statistics. A recent analysis of this relation, based on studies that made use of a wide range of sampling methods, sampled different populations and recorded numbers of different sexual partners over differing time intervals (ranging from the previous month to lifetime), revealed a linear relation on a logarithmic scale with coefficient values $a = 0.555$, $b = 3.231$ (Anderson & May 1988). Why there should be such a tight relation between the two statistics, irrespective of sampling method and sample population, is unclear at present (figure 1). However its existence enables us to express (2) in the form

$$c = m + am^{b-1}. \tag{4}$$

A summary of the mean rates of sexual partner change recorded in studies of male homosexual communities in the U.K. is presented in table 4.

The focus in models of HIV transmission on the rate of sexual partner change glosses over

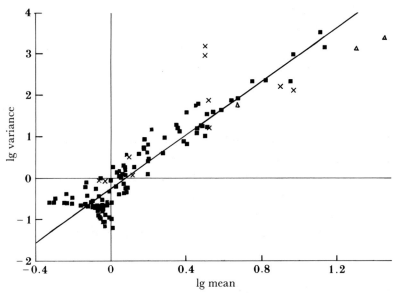

FIGURE 1. A scatter plot of the logarithm (base 10) of the variance in a reported number of different sexual partners against the logarithm of the mean number of sexual partners, from a wide range of published and unpublished studies (see Anderson & May 1988). The solid line denotes the best fit power model of the form defined by equation (4) in the main text. The squares record data from studies of heterosexuals in developed countries, the crosses are data from studies of homosexual males and the triangles are from studies of heterosexuals in developing countries.

TABLE 4. NUMBER OF SEXUAL PARTNERS PER TIME UNIT

(n = sample size)

population	n	time unit	mean number of partners — mean	median	reference
heterosexual and general					
U.K. (m+f), BMRB	—	per year	0.92	—	Anderson (1988)
U.K. (m+f), Harris poll	823	per year	1.50	—	Anderson (1988)
U.K. Students (m+f)	41	per year	1.50	—	Anderson (1988)
U.S.A. (m+f)	346	past year	6.3		Fischl et al. (1988)
		past 5 years	14.9	—	Fischl et al. (1988)
U.S.A. (m+f)	851	past 3 months	1.49		Baldwin & Baldwin (1988)
		past year	2.11		Baldwin & Baldwin (1988)
U.S.A. (m)	—	1985	2.84	—	Guydish & Coates (1988)
		1987	1.7	—	Guydish & Coates (1988)
African (m+f)	84	lifetime	7.5	—	Cornet et al. (1988)
Zaire, AIDS (m)	20	past year	7	—	Piot et al. (1984)
Zaire, AIDS (f)	18	past year	3	—	Piot et al. (1984)
Zaire, HIV+ couples	257	per year	5.5	—	Nzila et al. (1988)
(f)	257	per year	1.0	—	Nzila et al. (1988)
rural Uganda (f)	126	past 5 years	1.2	—	Hudson et al. (1988)
10–14	24	past 5 years	0.3	—	Hudson et al. (1988)
15–19	19	—	0.8	—	Hudson et al. (1988)
20–34	51	—	1.5	—	Hudson et al. (1988)
35–49	21	—	1.0	—	Hudson et al. (1988)
50+	11	—	0.5	—	Hudson et al. (1988)
rural Uganda (m)					
10–14	23	—	1.0	—	Hudson et al. (1988)
15–19	19	—	3.8	—	Hudson et al. (1988)
20–34	42	—	2.8	—	Hudson et al. (1988)
35–49	20	—	3.5	—	Hudson et al. (1988)
50+	19	—	1.9	—	Hudson et al. (1988)

TABLE 4. *(Cont.)*

population	n	time unit	mean number of partners		reference
			mean	median	
East African pastoralist (m)	132	per year	11.8	—	Konings *et al.* (1989)
Rwanda (m)	27	per year	3.0	—	Van De Perre *et al.* (1985)
female partners of bisexual men					
U.S.A.	169	past 2 years	2.9	—	Winkelstein *et al.* (1986)
U.S.A.	123	past 6 months, 1984	2.81	—	Winkelstein *et al.* (1987)
		past 6 months, 1986	1.81	—	Winkelstein *et al.* (1987)
Brazil HIV+	45	past 2 years	3.0	—	Costa *et al.* (1988)
Brazil HIV−	133	past 2 years	3.0	—	Costa *et al.* (1988)
male homosexual partners					
U.K.	100	per month 1984/5	4.7	3	Carne *et al.* (1987)
		per month 1986	—	1	Carne *et al.* (1987)
U.K. BMRB	—	per year	8.7	—	Anderson (1988)
	156	per 3 months	3.0	—	Anderson (1988)
		per year	10.5	—	Anderson (1988)
	298	per 3 months	3.7	—	Anderson (1988)
		per year	8.7	—	Anderson (1988)
	284	per 3 months	3.1	—	Anderson (1988)
		per year	7.1	—	Anderson (1988)
	251	per 3 months	2.0	—	Anderson (1988)
		per year	4.8	—	Anderson (1988)
Northern Ireland	30	per year 1984	16.6	—	Maw *et al.* (1987)
		per year 1985/6	20.8	—	Maw *et al.* (1987)
Belgium	526	1984	14.4	—	Goilav *et al.* (1988)
		1986	12.2	—	Goilav *et al.* (1988)
Netherlands	940	past 6 months	19.1	—	Countinho *et al.* (1987)
Italy	75	per month	—	10	Tirelli *et al.* (1988)
U.S.A. SF	655	1982	3.7	—	McKusick *et al.* (1985)
U.S.A. SF	454	1983	3.2	—	McKusick *et al.* (1985)
U.S.A. SF (steady)	126	1978	1.6	—	CDC (1987)
		1984	2.5	—	CDC (1987)
		1985	1.5	—	CDC (1987)
U.S.A. SF (non-steady)	126	past 4 months 1978	29.3	16	CDC (1987)
		past 4 months 1984	14.5	3	CDC (1987)
		past 4 months 1985	5.5	1	CDC (1987)
U.S.A.	78	per year	—	27	Jaffe *et al.* (1983)
U.S.A.	42	per year	—	25	Jaffe *et al.* (1983)
U.S.A. Kaposi's sarcoma and PCP patients	50	per year	61	—	Jaffe *et al.* (1983)
U.S.A. aware of HIV status	670	past 6 months	3.5	—	Fox *et al.* (1987)
U.S.A. unaware of HIV status	331	past 6 months	3.9	—	Fox *et al.* (1987)
U.S.A. NY	745	per year, pre 1985	—	36	Martin (1987)
		1985	8	—	Martin (1987)
U.S.A. Chicago	637	per month	1.74	—	Joseph *et al.* (1987)
U.S.A. Madison	488	past month 1982	6.2	—	Golubjatanikov *et al.* (1983)
		past month 1983	3.2	—	Golubjatanikov *et al.* (1983)
U.S.A. MACS HIV+	95	past 6 months	10	—	Kingsley *et al.* (1987)
		past 2 years	—	36	Kingsley *et al.* (1987)
		lifetime	—	200	Kingsley *et al.* (1987)
U.S.A. MACS HIV−	2412	past 6 months	—	5	Kingsley *et al.* (1987)
		past 2 years	—	20	Kingsley *et al.* (1987)
		lifetime	—	100	Kingsley *et al.* (1987)

TABLE 4. (*Cont.*)

population	n	time unit	mean number of partners		reference
			mean	median	
Brazil HIV+	45	past 2 years	—	30	Costa *et al.* (1988)
HIV—	133	past 2 years	—	10	Costa *et al.* (1988)
customers of prostitutes					
Rwanda (m)	25	per year	—	31	Van De Perre *et al.* (1985)
prostitutes (f)					
U.S.A. NY	78	past year	256	200	Seidlin *et al.* (1988)
Netherlands	117	per month	84	—	Van den Hoek *et al.* (1988)
Brazil	113	per year	800	—	Castello-Branco *et al.* (1988)
Kenya	429	per day 1985	3.7	—	Plummer *et al.* (1988)
HIV+	261	per day 1985	3.8	—	Plummer *et al.* (1988)
HIV—	168	per day 1985	3.6	—	Plummer *et al.* (1988)
using oral contraceptive	120	per day 1985	4.0	—	Plummer *et al.* (1988)
not using oral contraceptive	309	per day 1985	3.5	—	Plummer *et al.* (1988)
highly educated	78	per day 1985/6	3.8	—	Plummer *et al.* (1988)
medium educated	82	per day 1985/6	3.9	—	Plummer *et al.* (1988)
low educated	205	per day 1985/6	5.7	—	Plummer *et al.* (1988)
Kenya	124	per day 1985/7	3.8	—	Plummer *et al.* (1988)
HIV+	83	per day 1985/7	4.1	—	Plummer *et al.* (1988)
HIV—	41	per day 1985/7	3.3	—	Plummer *et al.* (1988)
Kenya low class	64	per year	963	—	Kreiss *et al.* (1986)
high class	26	per year	124	—	Kreiss *et al.* (1986)
Kenya HIV+	5	per month 1981	180	—	Piot *et al.* (1987)
Kenya HIV+	70	per month 1984/5	123	—	Piot *et al.* (1988)
HIV—	111	per month 1981	54	—	Piot *et al.* (1988)
HIV—	57	per month 1984/5	117	—	Piot *et al.* (1988)
Zaire	377	past week	3.7	—	Mann *et al.* (1988)
		past month	15.9	—	Mann *et al.* (1988)
		past year	158.0	—	Mann *et al.* (1988)
		lifetime	703.0	—	Mann *et al.* (1988)
HIV+	—	lifetime	—	600	Mann *et al.* (1988)
HIV—	—	lifetime	338	—	Mann *et al.* (1988)
Nigeria	823	per day	3.3	—	Mohammed *et al.* (1988)
Nigeria	35	per month	—	3.0	Ayoola *et al.* (1988)
Nigeria	767	per day	3.3	—	Chikwem *et al.* (1988)
		per year	1046	—	Chikwem *et al.* (1988)
Rwanda	33	per month	—	44	Van De Perre *et al.* (1985)
Somalia	55	per week	14	—	Jama *et al.* (1987)
prostitutes (m)					
Italy, IV drug	27	per month	—	50	Tirelli *et al.* (1988)
Italy, IV drug	76	per month	—	100	Tirelli *et al.* (1988)
Brazil	24	per year	10	—	Castello-Branco *et al.* (1988)
Brazil, transvestites	16	per year	480	—	Castello-Branco *et al.* (1988)
STD patients					
Canada (f)	707	past year	—	12	Elmslie *et al.* (1988)
Kenya (f)	40	past year	17	—	Kreiss *et al.* (1986)
Kenya (f), HIV+	8	per month	1.2	—	Piot *et al.* (1987)
Kenya (f), HIV—	113	per month	1.2	—	Piot *et al.* (1987)
Kenya (m), HIV+	36	per month	1.5	—	Piot *et al.* (1987)
Kenya (m), HIV—	232	per month	1.1	—	Piot *et al.* (1987)
Kenya (m)	115	past 6 weeks	1.7	—	Greenblatt *et al.* (1988)
Kenya (m), HIV+	19	past 6 weeks	1.4	—	Greenblatt *et al.* (1988)
Kenya (m), HIV—	96	past 6 weeks	1.8	—	Greenblatt *et al.* (1988)

much detail concerning variability in type of sexual activity between partnerships (e.g. oral or anal sex, etc.). Extensive studies of a large cohort of 4955 homosexual and bisexual men from the Baltimore, Chicago, Los Angeles and Pittsburgh areas of the U.S.A. (the Multicentre AIDS Cohort Study (MACS)) that started in 1983, revealed that the number of different sexual partners is, overall, the most important factor in determining the likelihood of HIV infection. However, among those with high rates of partner change, other factors such as the frequency of receptive and insertive anal intercourse are of great significance (Ginzburgh *et al.* 1988). A total of 8% of the 2915 individuals who were seronegative at the start of the study acquired infection over a two-year period. The rate of seroconversion among men who reported practising receptive but not insertive anal intercourse was 3.6 times higher than among men practising insertive intercourse alone, despite reports of 38% more different partners among those who practised insertive intercourse only.

(f) Changes in sexual behaviour

Education and a knowledge of the devastating impact of HIV infection, via friendship and association with infected individuals, has resulted in significant changes in sexual behaviour among male homosexuals in countries such as the U.S.A. and the U.K. Evidence for such changes comes indirectly from a decline in the incidences of other sexually transmitted infection such as gonorrhoea (Carne *et al.* 1986; Gellan & Ison 1986), and directly from longitudinal surveys of rates of sexual partner change, type of sexual activity and the frequency of practice of 'safe-sex' methods (Ginzburgh *et al.* 1988). Personal acquaintance with someone who has AIDS appears to be a powerful motivator for a change in sexual behaviour.

Unfortunately, no single study has charted changes in rates of sexual partner change, year by year, over the course of the epidemic. One study at four different sampling time points between February 1986 and January 1987 in the U.K. revealed a 50% reduction in claimed rates of partner change over the one-year time interval (see figure 2 and BMRB (1987)). More generally, however, the degree to which habits have changed in the male homosexual community in the U.K. from 1978 to the present, remains a matter of speculation (Evans *et al.* 1989). Reported declines in the incidences of other sexually transmitted diseases among male homosexuals suggest changes in behaviour were beginning to have an impact on disease

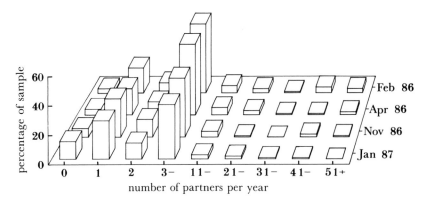

FIGURE 2. Patterns of change in the frequency distribution of reported numbers of different sexual partners per year in samples of male homosexuals in England drawn in February (10.5), April (8.7) and November 1986 (7.1) and January 1987 (4.8) (data from BMRB 1987). The mean rate of partner change per annum declined from 10.5 in February 1986 to 4.8 in January 1987.

transmission in the early 1980s (Weller *et al.* 1984; Johnson & Gill 1989; Loveday *et al.* 1989). It must be stressed, however, that accurate prediction of future trends in the incidence of AIDS in male homosexuals requires a quantitative understanding of temporal changes in sexual behaviour.

3. MATHEMATICAL MODELS

The general model of HIV transmission dynamics in a one-sex population with heterogeneity in sexual activity is essentially that first proposed by Anderson *et al.* (1986),

$$\frac{\partial x(s, t)}{\partial t} = \Lambda(s, t) - [\lambda(s, t) \, s + \mu] \, x(s, t), \tag{5}$$

$$\frac{\partial y(u, s, t)}{\partial t} + \frac{\partial y(u, s, t)}{\partial u} = - [v(u) + \mu] \, y(u, s, t), \tag{6}$$

with boundary and initial conditions:

$$x(s, t_0) = \Lambda(s, t_0)/\mu, s > 0, \tag{7}$$

$$y(0, s, t) = \lambda(s, t) \, sx(s, t), t > t_0, \tag{8}$$

$$y(u, s, t_0) = \eta(u, s), \tag{9}$$

where

s = sexual activity (new partners per unit time),

t = time,

t_0 = time at which infected person(s) entered the population,

$\int_a^b x(s, t) \, \mathrm{d}s$ = number of uninfected people with activity between a and b, at time t,

$\int_c^d \int_a^b g(u, s, t) \, \mathrm{d}s \, \mathrm{d}u$ = number of infected people with activity between a and b, who become infected between times $t-c$ and $t-d$, at time t,

$\Lambda(s, t)$ = rate of recruitment of newly sexually active people to the uninfected population, with activity s, at time t. The activity of an individual does not change with time,

μ = reciprocal of average duration of a sexual 'lifetime',

u = time since becoming infected,

$v(u)$ = fractional loss rate, per unit time, of individuals who have been infected for a time u. Losses occur as individuals develop AIDS. The hazard function $v(u)$ is

[19]

related to the probability density function for the incubation period of AIDS, $f(u)$, by

$$f(u) = v(u) \exp\left\{-\int_0^u v(x)\, dx\right\},\tag{10}$$

$\int_c^d \int_a^b \eta(u,s)\, ds\, du =$ the initial number of infected people (i.e. at $t = t_0$), with activity between a and b, who have been infected for a time between c and d,

$\lambda(s,t)\, s =$ fraction per unit time of uninfected people with activity s who become infected at time t (the so-called force of infection). For variable infectiousness, we write

$$\lambda(s,t) = \int_0^\infty \rho(s,r,t)\, \frac{\displaystyle\int_0^\infty \beta(u)\, y(u,r,t)\, du}{\displaystyle x(r,t) + \int_0^\infty y(u,r,t)\, du}\, dr,\tag{11}$$

where

$\beta(u) =$ infectiousness of someone who has been infected for a time u, i.e. the probability per unit, time of being infected through sexual contact with such a person. Note that if $\beta(u)$ is a constant β, then $\lambda(s,t)$ reduces to the integral of $\rho(s,r,t)$ times the fraction of people with activity r who are infectious (at time t), times β,

$\rho(s,r,t) =$ the fraction of the partners which someone of activity s taken among people with activity r, i.e. the 'contact function'.

Note that in this formulation, no account is taken of the number of times sexual intercourse occurs between partners.

We now outline some specific details of the model, and certain approximations that facilitate numerical analysis.

(a) Recruitment

We approximate the recruitment function $\Lambda(s,t)$ by the function $\Lambda W[s, a(t), b(t)]$, where Λ is the total number of sexually active individuals entering the susceptible population per unit time, and W is a Weibull probability density function describing the distribution of sexual activity of these recruits:

$$W(s, a(t), b(t)) \equiv b(t)\, a(t)^{b(t)} s^{b(t)-1} \exp\{-(a(t)\, s)^{b(t)}\}.\tag{12}$$

The mean and variance of the sexual activity of recruits is therefore given by:

$$m(t) = \frac{1}{b(t)}\, \Gamma\left(1 + \frac{1}{b(t)}\right)\tag{13}$$

and

$$\mathrm{var}\,(t) = m(t)\left[\frac{1}{\dfrac{\Gamma(2 + b(t) - 1)}{\Gamma^2(1 + 1/b(t))}}\right]\tag{14}$$

[20]

respectively, where $\Gamma(x)$ is the gamma function

$$\Gamma(x) = \int_0^\infty u^{x-1}\,e^{-u}\,du. \tag{15}$$

We simplify matters somewhat by assuming that the empirical relation between mean and variance of sexual activity described earlier (see Anderson & May 1988) holds true, so that (see equation (3)):

$$\text{var}(t) = a\,m(t)^b. \tag{16}$$

We can then treat W as a function with one parameter only, by taking a given mean activity $m(t)$, calculating var (t) from (16), and using (13) and (14) to obtain the approximate values of $a(t)$ and $b(t)$. We therefore use the shorthand notation $W[s, m(t)]$.

(b) Incubation period and infectiousness

Major reductions in the computations associated with solving the model can be made by careful choice of $f(u)$ and $\beta(u)$ (see Blythe & Anderson 1988 a, b). We express the incubation period probability density function as the sum of three exponential terms:

$$f(u) = \sum_{j=1}^3 a_j \exp(-\sigma_j u), \quad j = 1, 2, 3, \tag{17}$$

where
$$a_j = \prod_{i=1}^3 \sigma_j \Big/ \prod_{\substack{i=1 \\ i \neq j}}^N (\sigma_i - \sigma_j), \quad j = 1, 2, 3, \tag{18}$$

and the σ_j are the reciprocals of the average duration of each exponentially distributed sub-stage. By assigning a fixed value β_j to each sub-stage, we may replace (10) by the set of three simple equations:

$$\frac{\partial y_1(s, t)}{\partial t} = \lambda(s, t)\,sx(s, t) - (\sigma_1 + \mu)\,y_1(s, t), \tag{19}$$

$$\frac{\partial y_i(t)}{dt} = \sigma_{j-1}\,y_{j-1}(s, t) - (\sigma_j + \mu)\,y_j(s, t), \quad j = 2, 3. \tag{20}$$

With initial conditions

$$y_1(s, t_0) = \int_0^\infty \eta(u, s)\,du, \tag{21}$$

$$y_j(s, t_0) = 0, \quad j = 2, 3, \tag{22}$$

making the simplifying assumption that the invading infected individuals are all in the initial infectious sub-stage.

The incidence of AIDS (rate at which new cases are diagnosed per unit time) is then

$$V(t) = \sigma_3 \int_0^\infty y_3(s, t)\,ds, \tag{23}$$

while we may write

$$\lambda(s, t) = \int_0^\infty \rho(s, r, t)\frac{\sum_{j=1}^3 \beta_j y_j(r, t)}{N(r, t)}\,dr, \tag{24}$$

where
$$N(r, t) = x(r, t) + \sum_{j=1}^3 y_j(r, t); \tag{25}$$

$\int_a^b N(r, t)\,dr$ is the total number of people with activity between a and b at time t.

[21]

Following Blythe & Anderson (1988b), we shall assume that the infectiousness of an individual is relatively high immediately after infection occurs ($\beta_1 > 0$), is effectively zero for a time ($\beta_2 = 0$), and rises again as a diagnosis of AIDS is approached ($\beta_3 > 0$).

(c) Contact function

The function $\rho(s, r, t)$ describes the mixing between individuals of different activity, and must satisfy the three constraints:

$$1 \geqslant \rho(s, r, t) \geqslant 0, s, r, t, \tag{26}$$

$$\int_0^\infty \rho(s, r, t) \, \mathrm{d}r = 1, \forall s, t, \tag{27}$$

$$sN(s, t) \rho(s, r, t) = rN(r, t) \rho(r, s, t), \forall s, r, t. \tag{28}$$

Equations (26) and (27) reflect the fact that ρ is effectively a probability density function, whereas (24) expresses the requirement that the total number of partnerships between s-people (i.e. those with activity s) and r-people must equal the total number of partnerships between r-people and s-people. It is expected that ρ must lie somewhere between two limiting cases. At one extreme, individuals (of any activity) take their partners at random from the population. In this case the activity level with the most number of partnerships (i.e. $rN(r, t)$) is most strongly represented, and ρ becomes a function of r and t alone, namely:

$$\rho(s, r, t) = \frac{rN(r, t)}{\displaystyle\int_0^\infty zN(z, t) \, \mathrm{d}z}. \tag{29}$$

This case is known as 'proportionate mixing'. An example of $\rho(s, r)$ (for constant population size $\int_0^\infty N(s) \, \mathrm{d}s$) is shown in figure 3$a$.

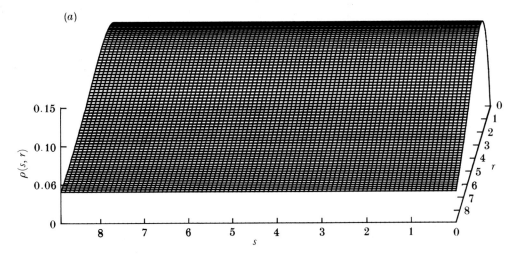

FIGURE 3. For legend see opposite.

[22]

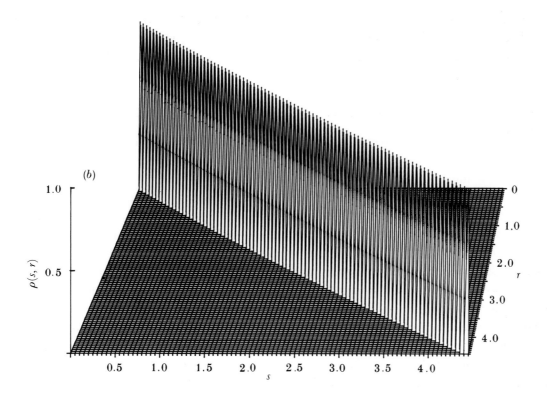

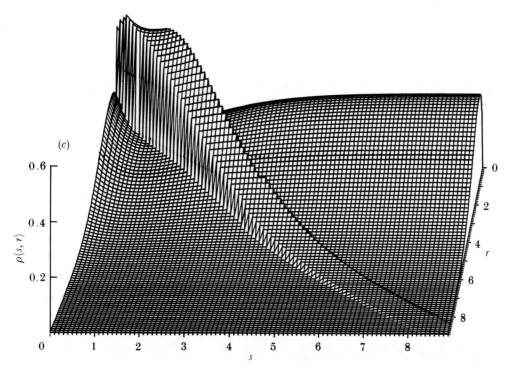

FIGURE 3. Contact functions. (*a*) The function $\rho(s, r, t)$ describes the mixing between individuals in different sexual activity classes. The case illustrated is for proportionate mixing where s and r denote the activity class of each individual in any given partnership (see text). (*b*) The extreme case where individuals only chose partners from their own activity level such that $\rho(s, r, t)$ becomes a delta function with $s = r$. (*c*) A mixture of proportionate mixing and preferred mixing within a given activity class (see Jacquez *et al.* 1988).

At the other extreme, individuals only select partners of their own activity level, so that $\rho(s, r, t)$ becomes a delta-function at $s = r$ (schematically represented in figure 3b). In this case (11) becomes:

$$\lambda(s, t) = \frac{\int_0^\infty \beta(u)\, y(u, s, t)\, \mathrm{d}u}{x(s, t) + \int_0^\infty y(u, s, t)\, \mathrm{d}u}, \tag{30}$$

so that there is no mixing between individuals from different activity levels. We do not believe that this case has any practical relevance. It simply serves to define the extreme case of preferential mixing.

The proportionate mixing solution has been used in a variety of situations (e.g. Barbour 1978; Nold 1980; Anderson & May 1984; Hethcote & York 1984; Dietz & Schenzle 1985; Anderson & Grenfell 1986; Hethcote & van Ark 1987; Blythe & Anderson 1988c; Castillo-Chavez $et\ al.$ 1988); while recently Sattenspiel (1987a, b); Sattenspiel & Simon (1988); Jacquez $et\ al.$ (1988) have explored alternative forms of mixing. Stanley (1989) and Blythe & Castillo-Chavez (1989) have also found new forms of ρ which satisfy the constraints given in equations (26)–(28) (figure 3c).

In this study we have not attempted to investigate the effects of preferential mixing, but instead chose to use the proportionate mixing model (equation (29)). Under these circumstances, we write:

$$\lambda(s, t) = \lambda(t) \equiv \int_0^\infty r \sum_{i=1}^3 \beta_i y_i(r, t)\, \mathrm{d}r \bigg/ \int_0^\infty r N(r, t)\, \mathrm{d}r. \tag{31}$$

(d) Aggregation approximation

Even in the simplified form resulting from the approximations outlined above, the transmission model still consists of three partial differential equations containing two integrals. To reduce the burden of computation further (which is advantageous if, for example, a sensitivity analysis is to be done), we introduce an extended version of Blythe & Anderson's (1988c) discretization scheme for the variable infectiousness model. This scheme is loosely related to the approximations of aggregation theory (see Iwasa 1987), and replaces the integro-partial differential equation system with a set of ordinary differential equations, whose behaviour should closely approximate that of the original system in defined ways (e.g. same steady states, stability properties, behaviour at $t \simeq t_0$, etc.).

Following Blythe and Anderson (1988c) we subdivide the continuum of sexual activity s into N discrete 'activity classes', with boundaries $\{s_i\}$, an ordered set with $s_{N+1} = 0$ and $s_{N+1} = \infty$, and characteristic levels of sexual activity $\{c_i\}$. The model system may then be written as

$$\mathrm{d}X_i(t)/\mathrm{d}t = \Lambda_i(\mathrm{t}) - [\lambda(t)\, c_i + \mu]\, X_i(t), \tag{32}$$

$$\mathrm{d}Y_{i,1}(t)/\mathrm{d}t = \lambda(t)\, c_i\, X_i(t) - (\sigma_1 + \mu)\, Y_{i,1}(t), \tag{33}$$

$$\mathrm{d}Y_{i,j}(t)/\mathrm{d}t = \sigma_{j-1}\, Y_{i,j-1}(t)\, (\sigma_j + \mu)\, Y_{i,j}(t), \tag{34}$$

for $i = 1, 2, \ldots, N$ and $j = 2, 3$, with initial conditions

$$X_i(t_0) = \Lambda_i(t_0)/\mu, \tag{35}$$

$$Y_{i,1}(t_0) = \int_{s_i}^{s_{i+1}} \int_0^\infty \eta(u, s)\, \mathrm{d}u\, \mathrm{d}s, \quad Y_{i,j}(t_0) = 0, \tag{36}$$

for $i = 1, 2, \ldots, N, j = 2, 3$. We have made the simplifying assumption that the initial infected individuals are all in the first infectious stage ($j = 1$). Equation (36) indicates that $Y_{j,1}(0) = $ constant. In addition we have:

$$\Lambda_i(t) = \int_{s_i}^{s_{i+1}} \Lambda(s, t) \, ds, \tag{37}$$

which is easily derived from (12)–(16), and

$$\lambda(t) = \frac{\sum\limits_{i-1}^{N} c_i \sum\limits_{j-1}^{3} \beta_j Y_{i,j}(t)}{\sum\limits_{i=1}^{N} c_i \left[X_i(t) + \sum\limits_{j=1}^{3} Y_{i,j}(t) \right]}. \tag{38}$$

Following Blythe & Anderson (1988c), the $\{c_j\}$ are chosen according to a scheme which is outlined below, with further details given in appendix A. $N-1$ of the $\{c_i\}$ are set in such a way as to give the same value for the steady-state susceptible class populations as for the equivalent section of the continuous s model, i.e.

$$X_i^* = \int_{s_i}^{s_{i+1}} x^*(s) \, ds, \quad i \neq i_B. \tag{39}$$

The remaining i_B^{th} class has an activity level c_{iB} set by requiring that the conditions for endemic persistence of infection is the same in the two models.

The addition of variable infectiousness adds little to the original scheme of Blythe & Anderson (1988c), but the change in sexual behaviour expressed in $\Lambda(s, t)$ introduces two complications.

(i) To reduce the complexity of the problem, we restrict changes in $\Lambda(s, t)$ to stepwise variation. Specifically, we use τ time intervals, each with a distinct value of mean sexual activity $m(t) = m_k$ ($k = 0, 1, \ldots, \tau$), and with boundaries $\{\tau_k = t\}$. Then for simplicity

$$\Lambda_{i,k}(t) = \Lambda \int_{s_i}^{s_{i+1}} W(s, m_k) \, ds = \Lambda \gamma_{i,k}, \; \tau_k \leqslant t < \tau_{k+1}. \tag{40}$$

(ii) We must take account of the non-trivial steady-state infected population when $m(t)$ becomes low enough such that the endemicity condition ($R_0(m) > 1$, see Blythe & Anderson 1988c) is violated. When this occurs, the scheme outlined above is inappropriate, as the infected steady-states are zero in both models (and $x^*(s) = N^*(s)$), such that the $\{c_i\}$ cannot be assigned values. In this case we use the simpler but less accurate approximation (Blythe & Anderson 1988c):

$$c_{i,k} = \int_{s_i}^{s_{i+1}} s\gamma(s, m_k) \, ds, \quad \tau_k \leqslant t < \tau_{k+1}. \tag{41}$$

(e) *Changes in the sexual behaviour of susceptible recruits to the sexually active population*

In the following sections (e), (f) and (g) we outline the methods adopted to simulate changes in sexual behaviour induced by education and a knowledge of the disease AIDS. Three types of behavioural changes are considered, namely changes in rates of sexual partner change among susceptible recruits to the sexually active adult population (e), changes in the magnitude of the average transmission probability β induced via the adoption of 'safer sex practices' (i.e. the use of condoms and a reduction in high-risk behaviours such as anal intercourse) (f) and changes in rates of sexual partner change among recruits and the sexually active population (g).

[25]

Changes in the distribution of rates of acquiring new sexually active population during the course of the epidemic are induced by defining a separate distribution for new susceptibles, with a reduced mean (from that prevailing in the existing sexually active population) and a variance as defined by the power law relationship given in equation (3). As detailed in section (d), the continuum of the sexually active is divided into N discrete activity classes, which are chosen to match those defined for the existing sexually active adults. At any given point in time the numbers of new recruits in each activity class are added to the identical activity class in the susceptible segment of the existing sexually active population. With a reduced mean level of activity, the system will eventually settle to a new equilibrium of endemic infection (with a reduced incidence of AIDS and a reduced prevalence of HIV infection) over many decades as the new recruits with reduced sexual activity gradually replace the existing population of higher activity, as they die from AIDS or natural causes.

(f) Reduction in transmission risk

It is relatively straightforward to incorporate an approximation to the effects of a decreasing prevalence of high-risk sexual practices, such as receptive anal intercourse. We simply let the $\{\beta_i\}$ themselves become (decreasing) functions of time $\{\beta_i(t)\}$. In order for the aggregation scheme of the previous section to be workable, we restrict the time-variation in the $\{\beta_i(t)\}$ to stepwise decreases coincident with the changes in the mean number of sexual partners, m_k. Hence we have:

$$\beta_j(t) = \beta_{j,k}, \quad \tau_k \leqslant t <, t_{k+1} \quad j = 1, 2, 3, \ k = 0, 1, \ldots, \tau, \tag{42}$$

and the final approximate form of the model is

$$dX_i(t)/dt = \Lambda \gamma_{i,k} - [\lambda_k(t) c_{i,k} + \mu] X_i(t), \tag{43}$$

$$dY_{i,1}(t)/dt = \lambda_k(t) c_{i,k} X_i(t) - (\sigma_1 + \mu) Y_{i,1}(t), \tag{44}$$

$$dY_{i,1}(t)/dt = \sigma_{j-1} Y_{i,j-1}(t) - (\sigma_j + \mu) Y_{i,j}(t) \tag{45}$$

$(j = 2, 3)$, with initial values given by (35) to (36), and

$$\lambda_k(t) = \frac{\sum\limits_{i=1}^{N} c_{i,k} \sum\limits_{j=1}^{3} \beta_{j,k} Y_{i,j}(t)}{\sum\limits_{i=1}^{N} c_{i,k} \left\{ X_i(t) + \sum\limits_{j=1}^{3} Y_{i,j}(t) \right\}}, \tag{46}$$

with the steps in $\{\gamma_{i,k}\}$, $\{c_{i,k}\}$ and $\{\beta_{i,k}\}$ occurring at times $\{\tau_k\}$, and the $\{c_{i,k}\}$ calculated according to the aggregation scheme of (43).

(g) Changes in the rate of acquiring new sexual partners within the existing sexually active population

Changes in the distribution of sexual activity within the population may be mirrored in a variety of ways. For example, individuals in different sexual activity classes within the susceptible (X) and infected (the Y_js) populations may be rearranged such that the activity within the total population conforms to a new distribution, $g'(i)$, dictated by a desired reduction in the mean activity and its associated variance (see (3)). So if $g_0(i)$ and $g_j(i)$ are the new distributions of activity for the susceptible and infected populations respectively, a set of solutions $\{g_j(i), j = 0, 1, 2, 3\}$ must be identified that satisfies the constraints:

$$g_0(i)\, X + \sum_{j=1}^{3} g_j(i)\, Y_j = g'(i)\, N, \tag{47}$$

$$X + \sum_{j=1}^{3} Y_j = N. \tag{48}$$

A number of solutions will satisfy these constraints and each can be translated into a particular programme of behavioural changes. For example, to satisfy a new mean and variance, changes may occur only in the susceptible population, or only among the infecteds. We consider four schemes in the results section of the paper. These are as follows.

(i) *Scheme* 1

If the probability of an individual moving to a particular sexual activity class (under a programme of change in behaviour) is independent both of the individual's infection status and of his current level of sexual activity, then the subpopulations will adopt identical distributions: $g_j(i) = g'(i), j = 0, 1, 2, 3$. As the initial distribution (before changes in behaviour) of activity among infecteds will contain (by definition) a larger than average number of individuals with high sexual activity, these 'random' changes between activity classes will result in a greater degree of change in behaviour among infecteds when compared with susceptibles.

If the probability of an individual moving to a particular sexual activity class is independent of infection status, but not of his current sexual activity, then it is necessary to make some assumptions concerning the dependence of the probability on sexual activity. We consider two possible sets of assumptions labelled schemes 2 and 3.

(ii) *Scheme* 2

We classify the sexual activity classes into those that receive individuals from other activity classes and those that lose individuals to other activity classes. We assume that individuals from the latter move into the former independent of infection status. Thus, if $G(i)$ is the gain and $L(i)$ the loss, from class i, if $G(i) > 0$, $L(i) = 0$ and if $G(i) = 0$, $L(i) > 0$, and $GX(i,j)$ is the gain to class i of susceptibles from class j, then

$$GX(i,j) = \left[G(i) \sum_{i=1}^{N} G(i) \right] [(X(j)/N(j))]\, L(j). \tag{49}$$

The movements are made to conform to a change in behaviour that reduces the mean level of activity by a defined amount and hence losses occur mainly in the high activity classes and gains mainly in the low-activity classes; consequently the effect of this scheme is a redistribution of individuals from the high-activity classes to the low-activity classes.

(iii) *Scheme* 3

Compared with scheme 2, scheme 3 minimizes the magnitude of individual behaviour change by permitting movements only between adjacent classes (except in the event that the adjacent class cannot supply the requisite number of individuals, when recourse must be made to the subsequent class). The direction of movement is always from a higher sexual activity class

[27]

into the adjacent lower-activity class, except when the loss required from the former exceeds the insufficiency of the latter, in which case, the excess is transferred to the adjacent higher class.

Thus we define a matrix v:

$$v(i,j) = 0,$$

$$w(i,j) = v(i-1,i) + G(i) - L(i) - \sum_{i+1}^{j-1} N_k,$$

if $w(i,j) > N_j$ then

$$v(i,j) = N_j,$$

$$v(j,i) = 0,$$

if $N_j > w(i,j) > 0$, then

$$v(i,j) = w(i,j),$$

$$v(j,i) = 0,$$

if $-L(i) < w(i,j) < 0$, then

$$v(i,j) = 0,$$

$$v(j,i) = -w(i,j),$$

if

$$w(i,j) < -L(i) \quad \text{then} \quad v(i,j) = v(j,i) = 0.$$

Then

$$GX(i,j) = X_j/N_j\, v(i,j). \tag{50}$$

(iv) *Scheme* **4**

If the probability of moving between sexual activity classes depends on an individual's infection status, then it is possible to restrict behaviour changes to a particular subpopulation (i.e. susceptibles or infecteds). An extreme case would be behavioural changes being restricted to the susceptible population such that:

$$g_0(i) = \left[g'(i)\, N - \sum_{j=1}^{3} Y_j(i)\right]\Big/ X, \tag{51}$$

where no change in activity occurs within the Y_j subpopulations. In principle, it is possible to confine behavioural changes to any particular group. However, if the group is small in size, relative to the total population, then it may not be possible to create sufficient changes in the target subpopulation to satisfy the desired degree of change (i.e. the desired reduction in the overall mean and its associated variance) in the total population. In those cases, it is necessary to dispense with the notion that the total sexually active population is redistributed as $g'(i)$. Instead, it is assumed that the group in question changes to adopt the new distribution $g'(i)$ with the overall distribution changing in a manner defined by the changes in the target group and their proportional representation in the total population.

4. MODEL PREDICTIONS

This section is divided into three parts: (*a*) a sensitivity analysis of model behaviour (particularly with respect to different parameter assignments for the set of transmission probabilities (the β_is) and the durations of the different infectiousness stages (the T_is); (b) the influence of changes in sexual behaviour and (c) the likely course of the epidemic in the male homosexual population of the U.K.

Certain parameters are assigned fixed values. The mean incubation period ($T = \sum T_i$) was set at eight years for sexually active adults (unless otherwise stated) in line with current estimates derived from studies of transfusion associated cases and cohorts of infected male homosexuals (Medley *et al.* 1988; Moss *et al.* 1989). With constant rates of joining and leaving the three infectious classes (Y_1, Y_2 and Y_3) and the AIDS class (A), the distribution of the incubation period is formed from the sum of three exponential distributions (see Blythe & Anderson 1988b). When the times (T_1, T_2 and T_3) spent in each of the three stages are 1, 4 and 3 years respectively (with $T = 8$ years), then the best fit Weibull distribution has a mean of 8.7 years, a variance of 5.92 and parameters $a_1 = 0.429$, $a_2 = 0.317$ (see Medley *et al.* 1988). The total number of male homosexuals in England and Wales was set at 500000 at the start of the epidemic (approximately 4 % of the sexually active male population between the ages of 16–46 years) (see Fay *et al.* 1989). The expected duration of sexual activity in the absence of HIV infection was set at 30 years ($1/\mu$). The net immigration rate of new susceptibles into the sexually active population, Λ, was set to satisfy the constraint that $\Lambda/\mu = 500000$. Immigration into the different sexual activity classes (the Λ_is) was determined by the power law relationship between the variance (σ^2) and mean (m) of the sexual activity distribution, as defined in (3), with coefficients $a = 0.555$, $b = 3.231$ (see Blythe & Anderson 1989). The proportion of infecteds, f, who eventually develop AIDS was fixed at 1.0 for all the numerical simulations. The mean rate of sexual partner change was fixed at 8.7 different partners per year with variance defined by (3) (see Blythe & Anderson 1988c). Six sexual activity classes were defined with annual rates of acquiring new partners of 0–2, 2–5, 5–10, 10–20, 20–50 and 50+. For illustrative purposes, the proportions in each of these activity classes, for a mean annual rate of partner change of 8.7 and a variance of 602 (as defined by (3) with coefficients $a = 0.555$, $b = 3.231$), are depicted in figure 4.

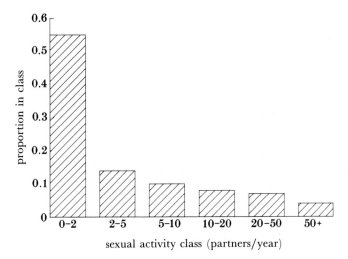

FIGURE 4. An illustration of the proportion of individuals in six sexual activity classes (0–2, 2–5, 5–10, 10–20, 20–50, 50+) (all defined as per year), for a distribution with mean, $m = 8.7$ and variance $\sigma^2 = 602$.

(*a*) *Sensitivity analysis*

(i) *Variation in the magnitude and duration of infectiousness*

As described earlier the model divides infected but non-AIDS individuals into three classes, Y_1, Y_2 and Y_3, with average durations of stay in each class of T_1, T_2 and T_3 respectively. The probability of transmission (i.e. infectiousness) is asumed to be constant within each class, but to vary between classes with values, β_1, β_2 and β_3 respectively for Y_1, Y_2 and Y_3. Individuals pass sequentially from class 1, via class 2 to class 3. They enter class 1 when first infected and leave class 3 when AIDS is diagnosed. The average incubation period of the disease, T, is thus $T = T_1 + T_2 + T_3$. The average duration of infectiousness, D, is the same as T provided each $\beta_i > 0$, if not D is equal to the sum of the stage durations in which $\beta_i > 0$. The basic reproductive rate of infection R_0, is simply

$$R_0 = c[\beta_1\,T_1 + \beta_2\,T_2 + \beta_3\,T_3], \tag{52}$$

given the assumption that the effective rate of sexual partner change, c, is the same for the three infected classes. We define the average transmission probability $\bar\beta$ over the average incubation period T as $\bar\beta = (\beta_1\,T_1 + \beta_2\,T_2 + \beta_3\,T_3)/T$.

In this subsection we examine the influence of changes in the values of the β_is and T_is on the pattern and magnitude of the epidemic. The first set of numerical simulations of the timecourse of the epidemic in the male homosexual population (simulation runs 1–9) employ three different values of the average transmission probability, $\bar\beta$, namely, 0.01, 0.05 and 0.1. For each value of $\bar\beta$ three different simulations were done with β_1 set at 0.01, 0.03 and 0.05, respectively. The parameter β_2 was set at zero in all simulations with the average infectious period fixed at 4 years with $T_1 = 1$ year, $T_2 = 4$ years and $T_3 = 3$ years, such that the average incubation period T was fixed at 8 years. The value of β_3 was adjusted for each value of β_1 such that the desired value of $\bar\beta$ (i.e. 0.01, 0.05 or 0.1) was obtained. A summary of the parameter values employed for each of the nine simulations is presented in table 5. With a fixed mean (8.7 year^{-1}) and variance (602.4) for the sexual partner change distribution (defined per year), and a fixed average infectious period (4 years), the $\bar\beta$ values of 0.01, 0.05 and 0.1 gave R_0 values of approximately 6, 30 and 61 respectively.

We summarize the results of these simulations by presenting, in graphical form, temporal changes (for a period of 100 years from the start of the epidemic) in the total number of HIV-infected persons (number seropositive), the proportion of infected individuals in the male homosexual community, the incidence of AIDS expressed per quarter year and the total population size of the community under the impact of the AIDS epidemic (from a starting size of 500 000 males at time $t = 0$). An example of these four variables plotted against time is provided in figure 5 for simulation run number 1 (see table 5 for parameter values). This particular case is one in which the magnitude of R_0 is set at 6.13 with an average transmission probability of 0.01 over the 8-year incubation period. The graphs ((*a*)–(*d*)) in figure 5 show the overall pattern of the epidemic in a community with high average rates of sexual partner change in which no change of behaviour occurs over the 100-year timespan. Note that the epidemic rises to a peak and then settles to a stable equilibrium which, for the parameter values employed in run 1 (see table 5), occurs about 50 years after the introduction of HIV. Also note that the peak in the number or proportion infected with HIV precedes that in the incidence of the disease AIDS because of the long and variable incubation period. Population size is depressed

TABLE 5. PARAMETER VALUES OF SIMULATION RUNS 1–9

simulation number	average incubation period T/years	infectious period average period/years	transmission probabilities				stage duration/years			*basic reproductive rate R_0	sexual activity classes (mean partner change in class/year)						*overall distribution mean variance	
			β	β_1	β_2	β_3	T_1	T_2	T_3		0–2 (0.55) 1	2–5 (0.14) 2	5–10 (0.1) 3	10–20 (0.08) 4	20–50 (0.07) 5	50+ (0.04) 6	m	σ_2
1	8	4	0.01	0.01	0	0.023	1	4	3	6.23	0.45	3.21	7.03	13.85	43.22	81.31	8.7	602
2	8	4	0.01	0.03	0	0.017	1	4	3	6.23	0.45	3.21	7.03	13.84	43.63	81.23	8.7	602
3	8	4	0.01	0.05	0	0.01	1	4	3	6.23	0.45	3.20	7.02	13.83	43.97	80.28	8.7	602
4	8	4	0.05	0.01	0	0.13	1	4	3	31.15	0.32	3.10	6.91	13.68	43.75	80.35	8.7	602
5	8	4	0.05	0.03	0	0.123	1	4	3	31.15	0.32	3.10	6.91	13.68	43.75	80.35	8.7	602
6	8	4	0.05	0.05	0	0.117	1	4	3	31.15	0.32	3.10	6.91	13.67	44.3	80.28	8.7	602
7	8	4	0.1	0.01	0	0.263	1	4	3	62.35	0.25	3.08	6.89	13.67	44.3	80.28	8.7	602
8	8	4	0.1	0.03	0	0.257	1	4	3	62.35	0.25	3.08	6.89	13.67	44.3	80.28	8.7	602
9	8	4	0.1	0.05	0	0.25	1	4	3	62.35	0.25	3.08	6.89	13.67	44.3	80.28	8.7	602

* Approximate values.

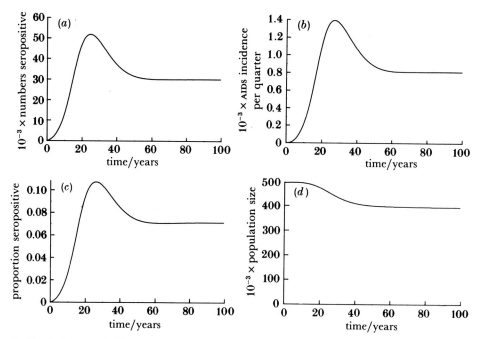

FIGURE 5. Simulation run 1. Temporal changes in (a) the number seropositive, (b) the quarter year incidence of AIDS, (c) the proportion seropositive in the population (= infected with HIV) and (d) the size of the population, as predicted by the model with parameter assignments as defined in run 1 in table 5.

from the disease-free level as a result of the mortality induced by AIDS, despite a constant rate of recruitment of new susceptible into the sexually active population.

A clearer picture of some of the details of the course of the simulated epidemic is displayed in figure 5 for run number 1. Graph (a) records changes through time in the numbers of individuals in each of the sexual activity classes (1–6) that record the rate of acquiring new sexual partners per year (see table 5). Snapshots at six time intervals are recorded for each sexual activity class. For a given class the left-hand bar denotes time zero and each subsequent bar denotes the numbers in that class at 10-year intervals (i.e. 0, 10, 20, 30, 40, 50 years). Note that mortality due to AIDS has the greatest proportional impact on those in the highest sexual activity class (6). After 50 years of the epidemic the numbers in this class are less than 30% of the size of the group at time $t = 0$. Also note that for the assigned parameter values for run number 1 the epidemic has little impact on activity class 1. Those with high rates of sexual partner change are both more likely to acquire infection and die from AIDS and to transmit it to others. In the early stages of the epidemic 71% of the total sexual partner changes in a given year are made by individuals in activity classes 5 and 6 who represent only 11% of the total population.

Graph (b) in figure 6 records changes through time in the proportion infected with HIV in each of the six sexual activity classes. Note that the increase in seropositivity is very rapid in the high activity class but very slow in the low activity class. In class 6 seropositivity attains a maximum value of around 80% whereas in class 1 seropositivity only rises to a few percent.

The shape and overall magnitude of the epidemic, the time interval between the start of the epidemic and the point of maximum disease incidence and the equilibrium incidence of disease and infection, depend on the magnitude of the basic reproductive rate R_0 and the values of its

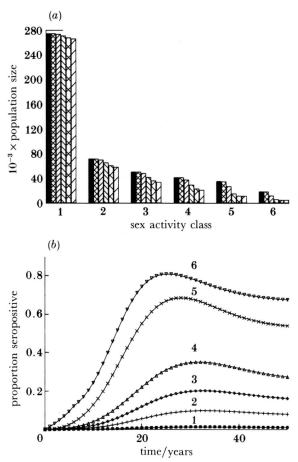

FIGURE 6. Simulation run 1. (a) Changes through time in the number of individuals in each of the six sexual activity classes (see main text). Snapshots at six time intervals are recorded for each activity class where the left-hand bar denotes time $t = 0$, and each subsequent bar denotes the numbers in that class at 10-year intervals, i.e. $t = 10, 20, 30, 40, 50$. (b) Changes through time in the proportion infected with HIV in each of the six activity classes.

component parameters (i.e. the β_is, T_is and c). Figure 7 illustrates the influence of the magnitude of the transmission probability during the first phase of infectiousness, β_1, on the shape of the epidemic, as represented by the incidence of AIDS (0.25 per year), for various values of R_0. In graphs (a), (b) and (c) the value of β_1 is set at 0.01, 0.03 and 0.05 respectively. In each graph the value of β_3 ($\beta_2 = 0$) is varied to give three different values of R_0, respectively 6 ($\bar{\beta} = 0.01$), 31 ($\bar{\beta} = 0.05$) and 62 ($\bar{\beta} = 0.1$). Note that the value of β_1 has a strong influence on the rate of increase in the epidemic over its early stages, and hence on the timing of peak incidence. High values of β_1 lead to rapid rises in incidence and an early peak, while low values lead to a less rapid rise and a later peak. The value of R_0, however, determines the overall magnitude of the epidemic and the level of the endemic equilibrium state (compare each of the three trajectories within each graph, see table 5 for parameter values). High values of R_0 result in rapid growth of the epidemic and it is more 'peaked' in character by comparison with that generated by lower values (figure 7). A clearer picture of the influence of the magnitude of β_1 on the rate of growth of the epidemic in its early phase is provided in figure 8 where the value of R_0 is held constant in each individual graph (6 in (a), 31 in (b) and 62 in (c)) and β_1 is varied

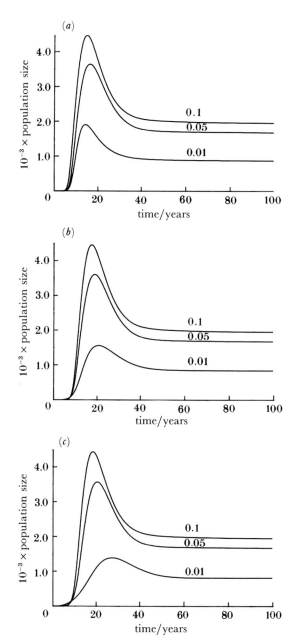

FIGURE 7. Temporal changes in the incidence of AIDS (defined per quarter year). In graph (a) the value of β_1 was held constant at 0.05 while the value of β_3 was varied to give β values of 0.1, 0.05 and 0.01 with $T_1 = 1$, $T_2 = 4$, $T_3 = 3$ (simulation runs 3, 6 and 9, in table 5). (b) Similar to (a) except that the value of β_1 was fixed at 0.03 (simulation runs 2, 5 and 8 in table 5).

from 0.01 to 0.05. The magnitude of β_1 in the first phase of infectiousness determines the rapidity with which the epidemic spreads, while the value of β_3 in the second phase of infectiousness helps to determine the magnitude of R_0, and hence the overall size of the epidemic (Anderson 1988a; May & Anderson 1988; Anderson & May 1988).

The rapidity of the rise in the incidence of AIDS reflects the rapid rise of the proportion infected with HIV in each of the six sexual activity classes. This is shown in figures 6b and 9. In both graphs the magnitude of R_0 was set at 6 but in figure 6b, β_1 was set at 0.01, and in

[34]

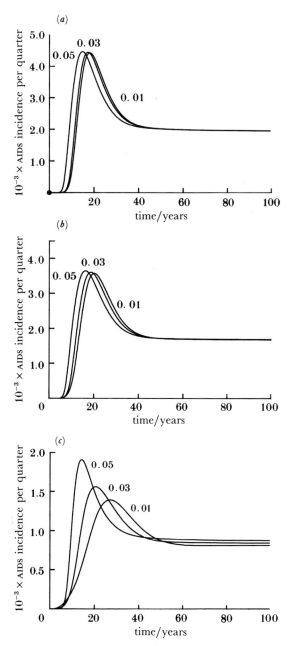

FIGURE 8. Temporal changes in the incidence of AIDS (defined per quarter year). In graph (a) the value of $\bar{\beta}$ was held constant at 0.1 while the value of β_1 was varied in 3 separate simulations with values of 0.01, 0.03 and 0.05 ($R_0 = 62.3$) (simulation runs 7, 8 and 9 in table 5). (b) Similar to (a) except that the value of $\bar{\beta}$ was fixed at 0.05 ($R_0 = 31.15$) (simulation runs 4, 5 and 6 in table 5).

figure 9, β_1 was set at 0.05 (run 3, see table 5). Note that with a high value of β_1 (0.05) for a fixed value of R_0 seroprevalence rises rapidly such that it attains a maximum value in the highest sexual activity class (6) 10 years after the start of the epidemic (figure 9). By contrast, for the low value of β_1 (0.01) the maximum proportion infected in class 6 occurs 20 years after the start of the epidemic (figure 6b). For higher values of R_0 (i.e. 31, with $\bar{\beta} = 0.05$, $\beta_1 = \beta_3 = 0.1$) the rapidity of rise in seroprevalence through time is even more marked (figure 10). The

[35]

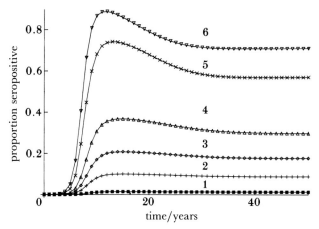

FIGURE 9. Temporal changes in the proportion infected with HIV (seropositive) in the six different sexual activity classes (1–6, see text). Parameter values were set as defined for simulation number 3 in table 5.

example recorded in figure 10 shows that HIV prevalence in the highest sexual activity class (6) again exceeds 90 % in around five years from the start of the epidemic (graph (*b*)) even though the prevalence in the total population only attains a maximum level of around 40 % 10–12 years after the start of the epidemic. This pattern is similar to that observed in male homosexuals attending sexually transmitted disease clinics in San Francisco in the U.S.A. in the period 1980–1985. For those with very high rates of sexual partner change seroprevalence rose from a few percent to around 90 % over the five-year period (Curran *et al.* 1988; CDC 1985). Broader-based surveys of prevalence of HIV infection in male homosexual communities in the U.S.A. in 1987–1988 suggest average prevalence levels of around 36 % (Curran *et al.* 1988; CDC 1988) about 10–12 years after the emergence of the epidemic in this risk group.

Also of interest in the simulated trajectories of the rise in the proportion of the population infected with HIV is the rate of change in the numbers or proportions infected during the course of the epidemic. As illustrated in figure 11 for simulation runs 4, 5 and 6, the rate of change in the numbers infected per quarter year rises rapidly in the early phase of the epidemic, declines in the middle phase, becomes negative just after the peak of the epidemic before settling to zero as the equilibrium state is reached. The nonlinear character of these changes is of particular importance. Note that before the peak in the numbers infected the rate of change begins to decrease quite markedly even in the absence of changes in sexual behaviour. This is a consequence of 'saturation' effects in the high sexual activity classes where, because of the high proportion infected, both partners in many sexual liaisons are already infected.

Observed longitudinal trends in the prevalence of HIV infection in populations of male homosexuals depend to some extent on the method employed to sample the population (Winkelstein *et al.* 1987). The study referred to above in San Francisco was based on homosexual/bisexual men recruited from sexually transmitted disease clinics in 1978 for ongoing studies of hepatitis B virus. A selected sample from this population who consented to blood tests in each year from 1978 to 1986 (i.e. a cohort study) revealed the trend recorded in figure 12 *a* (sample size 283 in 1978; CDC 1988). Prevalence again rose rapidly over the time interval 1980–1985, and plateaued at around 60 % by 1986. By way of a contrast, a non-cohort study of homosexual/bisexual men attending a sexually transmitted disease clinic in London showed a rapid rise in seroprevalence from 1981 to 1983 but thereafter the percentage of

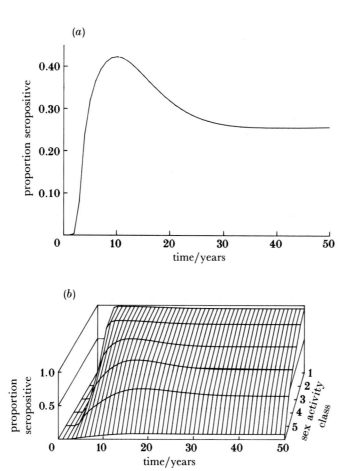

FIGURE 10. Temporal changes in the proportion infected with HIV (seropositive) (a) in the total population and (b) in the six different sexual activity classes (1–6). Parameter values: $R_0 = 31$, $\bar{\beta} = 0.05$, $\beta_1 = \beta_3 = 0.1$, $T_1 = 1$, $T_2 = 4$, $T_3 = 3$.

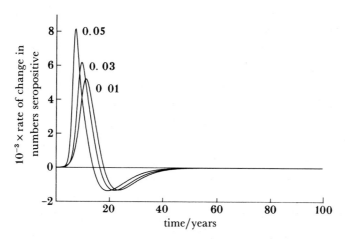

FIGURE 11. Temporal changes in the rate of change (per quarter year) in the numbers seropositive for HIV. Trends through time are recorded for simulation runs 4, 5 and 6 in table 5 (β values of 0.01, 0.03 and 0.05).

infected attendees at the clinic plateaued at around 25% (Carne *et al.* 1987; HMSO 1988) (figure 12*b*). In both cases the attained of a plateau was in part due to saturation effects and in part because of changes in sexual behaviour. This latter explanation is thought to be a major factor contributing to the relative low percentage infected in the London study, in comparison with that in San Francisco. The epidemic started later in London and hence a knowledge amongst homosexuals of what was occurring in the U.S.A. is believed to have stimulated changes in sexual behaviour at an earlier stage in the epidemic by comparison with that in San Francisco.

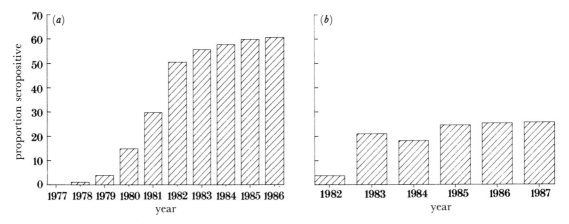

FIGURE 12. Temporal trends in the proportion seropositive for HIV recorded in two studies of groups of male homosexuals attending sexually transmitted disease clinics (*a*) in San Francisco, U.S.A. and (*b*) in London, U.K. The data in (*a*) are from table 12 in CDC (1987) and those in (*b*) are from Carne *et al.* (1987), table A 3.1 in HMSO (1988) and from Loveday *et al.* (1989). See source references for details of the study populations.

(ii) *Variation in the length of the non-infectious stage,* T_2

Changes in the average duration of the non-infectious period, T_2, between the two peaks in infectiousness can have a significant influence on the pattern of the epidemic. This point is illustrated in figure 13 where the magnitude of T_2 is varied (with values of 3, 4, 5 and 10 years) while β_1 and β_3 are held constant with values of 0.03 and 0.0167, respectively. Keeping β_1 and β_3 constant with fixed values of T_1 (1 year) and T_3 (3 years) constrains the magnitude of R_0 to the constant value of 6.2, irrespective of the value of T_2 (provided $\beta_2 = 0$). The epidemic is smaller in magnitude, is less 'peaked' in character and the equilibrium incidence of AIDS is lower when the value of T_2 is high, compared with lower values. This is in part a consequence of the long drawn out nature of the epidemic such that with long non-infectious periods a significant fraction of those infected in the early stages of the spread of infection (i.e. those in the high sexual activity classes) will have either died from natural causes or ceased sexual activity before progressing to the second phase of infectiousness.

(*b*) *Changes in sexual behaviour during the course of the epidemic*

Beneficial changes in sexual behaviour may occur via a reduction in the rate of acquiring new sexual partners (i.e. a change in the values of *m* and σ^2) or via an increase in the frequency of adoption of what are termed 'safer sex practices' (changes in the β_is). The latter include the use of condoms and a reduction in high risk behaviours such as anal sex. Such changes can be

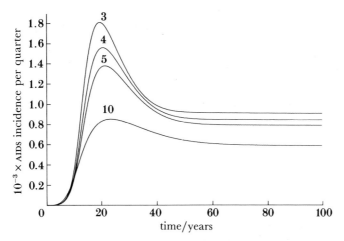

FIGURE 13. The effect of varying the duration of the non-infectious period (of length T_2 years) between the two periods of infectiousness on the predicted temporal trend in the incidence of AIDS (per quarter year). Four simulations are plotted with the value of R_0 held constant at 6.2 and the value of T_2 varied in the separate simulations to 3, 4, 5 and 10 years ($T_1 = 1$ year, $T_2 = 3$ years).

mirrored in the model in various ways. As described in the methods section of the paper we examine three different methods of representing changes in behaviour. These are: (i) reductions in the average rate of sexual partner change (m) among susceptible recruits to the sexually active population, via education at schools; (ii) reduction in the magnitudes of the transmission probabilities (the β_is) to mirror the adoption of 'safer sex practices' and (iii) reduction in the average rate of sexual partner change among recruits and the sexually active population via education in the general population and at schools.

(i) *Change in the rate of acquisition of new sexual partners among susceptible recruits to the sexually active population*

Changes in the behaviour of new recruits to the sexually active population (the Λ_is) were simulated in two different ways. In the first type of simulation, the mean rate of sexual partner change of the susceptible, recruits was reduced by a defined amount from 1983 onwards (the epidemic was assumed to have started in 1979, hence $t = 0$ in all simulations denotes 1979, $t = 10$ denotes 1989, etc.). Those recruited before 1983 and those sexually active before this date were assumed not to change their behaviour. In five different simulations, the mean rate of partner change, m (with the variance σ^2 calculated from the power low relation, see figure 1), was changed from 8.7 per year in the interval 1979–1983, to 6, 5, 4, 3 and 2 (all per year) from the beginning of 1983 onwards, respectively. The impact of such changes on the quarter-yearly incidence of AIDS is depicted in figure 14a for each of the five simulations. For comparison the incidence of AIDS in the absence of any behavioural change is also plotted against time. The parameter set used to generate these trajectories, aside from the differing assumptions concerning the mean rate of sexual partner change, m, were as defined for simulation run number 2.

In the second type of simulation the mean rate of acquiring sexual partners by new susceptible recruits to the sexually active population was reduced in a stepwise manner from 8.7 per year in 1979–1983, by one unit in each successive year up to 1988 (i.e. mean rates of sexual partner change of 7 per year in 1983, 6 per year in 1984, 5 per year in 1985, 4 per year

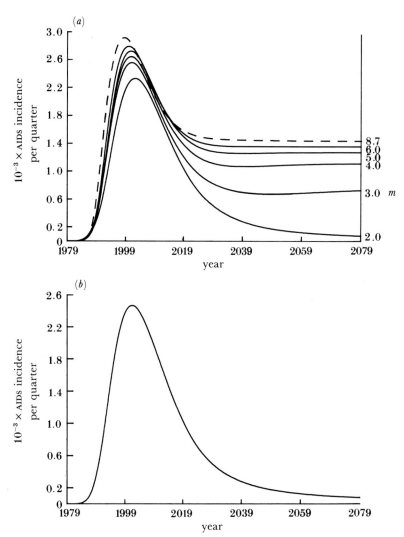

FIGURE 14. The impact of changes in sexual behaviour (reductions in the rate of acquisition of new sexual partners) among susceptible recruits to the sexually active population (with no change in behaviour among individuals in the sexually active population at the time point when changes in behaviour were initiated amongst the recruits). In (a) five simulations are recorded in which the mean rate of sexual partner change per year of recruits was reduced in 1983 (and thereafter) to 6.0, 5.0, 4.0, 3.0 and 2.0. The simulation for no change ($m = 8.7$ per year) is also plotted to provide a point of reference. Parameter values were set as defined by simulation run number 2 in table 5. In (b) the parameter values were as defined for (a) except that the mean rate of sexual partner change among new recruits was reduced in a step-wise manner from 8.7 per year in 1979–1983 by one unit in each success year up to 1988 (i.e. mean rates of 7 per year in 1983, 6 per year in 1984, 5 per year in 1985, 4 per year in 1986, 3 per year in 1987 and 2 per year from 1988 onwards).

in 1986, 3 per year in 1987 and 2 per year from 1988 onwards). Temporal changes in the quarter yearly incidence of AIDS under this pattern of change in behaviour is presented in figure 14b.

An assessment of the patterns recorded in figure 14 suggests that if the mean rate of partner change of the recruits is lowered significantly (i.e. from 8.7–2.0 in 1983) after the initial epidemic, the infection will die out in the population over a timespan of many decades (figure 14a). If the reduction is insufficient to reduce the overall basic reproductive rate, R_0, below unity in value, the behavioural change among new recruits will simply act to lower the level of the endemic equilibrium incidence of disease. Overall, the reductions in the total number of AIDS cases induced by these changes are limited in nature, by comparison with the trajectory displayed for the simulation in which no changes occur (figure 14 a). In other words, changes in the behaviour of the new recruits to the sexually active population are insufficient by themselves to have a marked impact on the initial epidemic of AIDS, before the attainment of the endemic equilibrium state. The reason for this is that, with a life expectancy of 30 years of sexual activity (in the absence of HIV infection), it takes a long period of time before the recruits (with their changed sexual behaviour) begin to constitute a majority of the sexually active population. Education must therefore be aimed at adults (the sexually active population) as well as teenagers (future recruits).

(ii) *Reductions in the transmission probability by the adoption of safe-sex practices*

Changes in behaviour via the adoption of 'safer sex' practices act to decrease the probability that the infection is transmitted during sexual contact between susceptible and infectious individuals. We simulated two different scenarios. In both cases changes in behaviour were assumed to reduce the values of the β_is by a similar amount (i.e. the overall value $\bar{\beta}$ was reduced by a defined amount). In the first type of scenario $\bar{\beta}$ was reduced to 0.75, 0.5 or 0.25 of its original value in different simulations. In separate simulations these changes were assumed to occur in 1983, 1986 and 1989. The results, expressed as temporal changes in the cumulative number of AIDS cases, are presented in figure 15. Three main points are illustrated by these numerical experiments. First, the proportional reduction in the total number of cases of AIDS is not equal to the proportional reduction in the magnitude of $\bar{\beta}$. Proportionally greater reductions in the cumulative number of cases of AIDS result from the larger reductions in $\bar{\beta}$ (i.e. a reduction of 75 % for example; figure 15). The second feature is the great benefit that accrues from changes in behaviour early in the course of the epidemic. Changes in 1983, for example, have a much more substantial impact than changes initiated in 1986 (figure 15 a, b). The final point of importance is that none of the proportional reductions in $\bar{\beta}$ are sufficient to reduce the magnitude of R_0 below unity. As such the infection persists and the cumulative number of cases of AIDS continues to grow over a timespan of many decades. For a large reduction in $\bar{\beta}$ the epidemic moves on an extremely long timescale.

The second type of simulation involved the cessation of transmission by setting $\bar{\beta} = 0$ at different time points in the course of the epidemic. Behavioural changes that blocked transmission were induced in separate simulations each year (1983–1989). The trajectories through time of the quarter year incidence of AIDS, and the total number of infected individuals, are recorded for each simulation in figure 16 a, b. The principle point illustrated by this simulation is the large number of AIDS cases that occur after the cessation of transmission as a direct result of the long and variable incubation period of the disease. Note that even if all transmission ceased in 1987, significant numbers of AIDS cases would still be reported over the subsequent 20-year period.

(iii) *Reductions in the rate of sexual partner change*

The third method of simulating changes in behaviour centres on changes in the probability distribution of the rate of acquiring new sexual partners per unit of time. Simulating such changes raises many complications in model formulation and requires careful definition of exactly how such changes are induced and who they influence. As described in the Methods

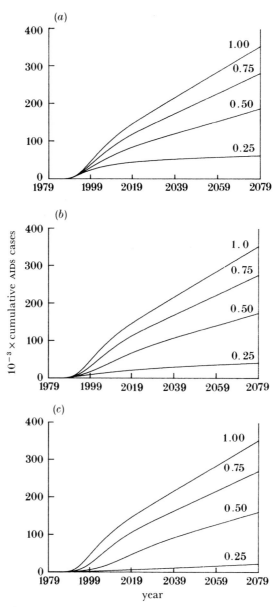

FIGURE 15. The influence of changes in the probability of transmission (β) induced by the adoption of safer-sex practices on the cumulative number of AIDS cases over a 100-year time span. The magnitude of $\bar{\beta}$ was reduced by 0.75, 0.5 and 0.25 of its pristine value in (a) 1989, (b) 1986 and (c) 1983 in separate simulations. Before the change the parameter values were as defined for simulation run number 2 in table 5. For a 25% reduction (in (a) 1989, (b) 1986 or (c) 1983) the parameter values were set at $\beta_1 = 0.0225$, $\beta_3 = 0.0125$, $R_0 = 4.6$. For a 50% reduction the values were set at $\beta_1 = 0.015$, $\beta_3 = 0.00835$, $R_0 = 3$ and for a 75% reduction the values were $\beta_1 = 0.0075$, $\beta_3 = 0.0042$, $R_0 = 1.5$. In all cases $T_1 = 1$, $T_2 = 4$, $T_3 = 3$ (years).

section we consider four schemes of behavioural change and examine their impact on the number of infected and the incidence of AIDS via simulations over a 100-year times period. For comparative purposes graphs denoting the outputs of separation simulation experiments also record temporal trends in the number infected or the incidence of AIDS under assumptions of no change and of changes restricted to the susceptible recruits to the active population.

The manner in which changes are induced (i.e. schemes 1–4) has a significant impact on the

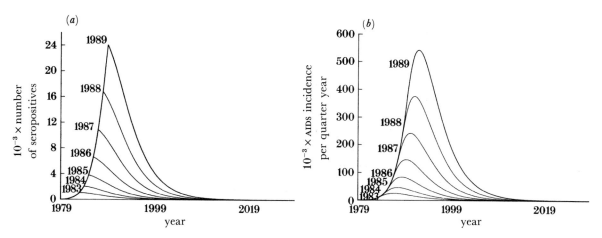

FIGURE 16. The influence of a cessation of transmission ($\bar{\beta} = 0$) induced at different time points (1983–1989) on the number of infected individuals in (a) (seropositives) and the incidence of AIDS per quarter year (b).

predicted temporal trends. In figure 17, for example, changes in the numbers infected are recorded for schemes 1–4 under the assumption that the mean rate of sexual partner change in the total population altered from 8.7 per year in the interval 1979 up to the end of 1988, to 5.0 per year from the beginning of 1989 onwards. In this particular example the changes made under schemes 1–4 satisfied the constraints defined in (47) and (48) (i.e. the mean rate of sexual partner change in the total population was 5.0 from the beginning of 1989 onwards). Under scheme 4, changes in behaviour were only induced in the susceptible population in 1989 and subsequent recruits who joined this subpopulation over the interval 1989–2079. Note that all the simulations converge to the same endemic state after many decades (except the situation where no behavioural change occurred). Also note that the greatest impact immediately

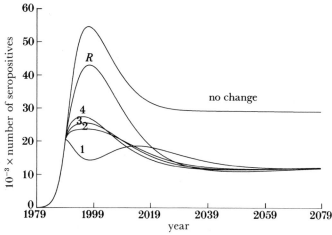

FIGURE 17. The influence of changes in the rate of sexual partner change in the sexually active population on the number of infecteds (seropositives). Various assumptions were made in different simulations concerning how the changes occurred and who they affected. As described in the text, four different schemes were simulated (labelled 1–4). A reduction in the mean rate of sexual partner change from 8.7 to 5.0 per year was made at the beginning of 1989 (parameter set as defined by simulation run number 2 in table 5). For reference the simulated trajectories for no change (labelled no change) and for changes in behaviour only among new recruits to the sexually active population (labelled R) are recorded in the graph.

[43]

following the instigation of the changes results from scheme 1 in which individuals move to new activity classes independent of infection status and past sexual activity. This pattern of 'random' movement induces the greatest change amongst the infected group since, on average, individuals in this subpopulation have higher rates of sexual partner change before the introduction of changes in behaviour. The induced change in behaviour via random reassortment from all classes of activity has the greatest impact on the average level of activity in this group and, as such, has the greatest immediate impact on the net rate of transmission within the population. The pattern of change in the incidence of AIDS under these assumptions are recorded in figure 18 *a*.

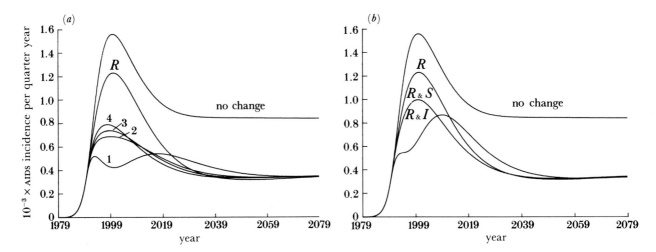

FIGURE 18. (*a*) The influence of a change in sexual behaviour among the sexually active population on the incidence of AIDS per quarter year. The different simulations and parameter sets are as defined in the legend to figure 17. (*b*) The influence of a change in behaviour (initiated in 1989) in particular infection subpopulations on the quarter yearly incidence of AIDS. As described in the text, the assumption made were as defined in scheme 4 in the methods section, where changes in behaviour are induced in particular infection subpopulations (R = susceptible recruits, S = sexually active susceptibles and I = sexually active infecteds (but not AIDS patients)), without making adjustments to satisfy the constraints defined in equations (49) and (48). At the beginning of 1989 the mean rate of partner change in a defined infection subpopulation was reduced from 8.7 to 5.0 per year (with associated changes in the variance as defined in equation (4)). The parameter set employed was as defined for simulation run number 2 in table 5.

The influence of a different pattern of changes in behaviour is recorded in figure 19 for scheme 4. In this example, changes in behaviour are induced in particular infection subpopulations only, without making adjustments to satisfy the constraints defined in (49) and (48) in the population as a whole (in contrast with scheme 4 in figure 17). The greatest impact is apparent when changes occur in the new recruits and the infected population (the mean rate of sexual partner change in the target subpopulation was reduced from 8.7 to 5.0 at the beginning of 1989). Changes in the numbers infected are recorded in figure 19 and changes in the incidence of AIDS are recorded in figure 18 *b*.

The general point illustrated by these different simulations is the importance, to the pattern of the epidemic, both of the manner in which behaviour changes and of the precise group influenced by such changes. Of the four schemes considered above, we believe that scheme 3 is more likely to reflect reality. This scheme is the most 'conservative' in the sense that changes are assumed to occur between adjacent classes of sexual activity. In other words, an overall

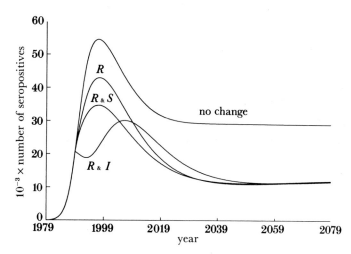

FIGURE 19. Identical to the simulations recorded in figure 18*b* but denoting the simulated changes through time in the number seropositive (parameter set number 2 in table 5).

reduction in the mean level of activity in the population occurs via individuals moving from their current activity class to the next lowest activity class.

So far we have only considered a single change in behaviour (a reduction in the mean from 8.7 to 5.0) occurring at one point in time, i.e. 1989). The timing of the change in behaviour, relative to the starting point of the epidemic (1979), has a significant impact on the overall magnitude of the epidemic. Adopting scheme 3, figure 20 records changes in the numbers infected (graph (*a*)) and the incidence of AIDS (graph (*b*)) for simulations in which the change in behaviour occurred at different time points, namely in 1983, 1985, 1987 and 1989. Note that all simulation converge after many decades on the same equilibrium point. Changes in behaviour early on in the epidemic (i.e. 1983) have a major impact on the number infected and the incidence of AIDS over the first two decades.

Substantial changes in sexual behaviour among the male homosexual community in England and Wales have occurred since the start of the AIDS epidemic, as illustrated in figure 2. The precise timing of these changes and their magnitudes is difficult to ascertain from current data. Two recent studies of HIV incidence and sexual behaviour in male homosexual communities in London and Amsterdam suggest that major changes in the rate of infection and pattern of behaviour occurred in these two populations around 1985–1986 (Evans *et al.* 1989; van Griesven *et al.* 1989). For example in the study of van Griesven *et al.* (1989) in Amsterdam, the incidence of HIV infection (defined as the percentage of the study cohort who acquired HIV per annum) increased sharply over the interval 1981–1984 and then fell markedly in the period 1985–1987 (figure 21). As illustrated by our numerical simulations (see figure 11) a rapid rise followed by a rapid fall in the incidence of new infections is to be expected, even in the absence of behavioural changes, because of saturation effects in the high activity classes. The studies in London and Amsterdam were to some extent focused on high activity classes (i.e. attendees at sexually transmitted disease clinics), but the behavioural data collected in these two surveys did suggest that significant changes in behaviour, both with respect to the frequency of high-risk activities plus rates of sexual partner change, did occur during the period 1986–1987. Unlike our earlier simulations, such changes have presumably occurred in a continuous manner since

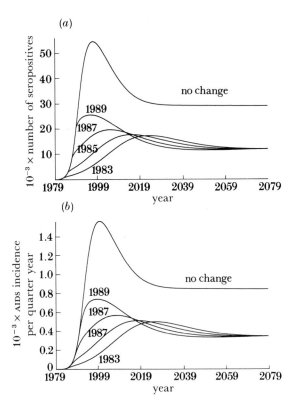

FIGURE 20. The influence of the timing of a change in sexual behaviour on temporal trends in the quarter yearly incidence of AIDS in (b) and the number infected (seropositive) in (a). In separate simulations a single alteration in behaviour, in which the mean rate of sexual partner change was reduced from 8.7 to 5.0 per year (with an associated change in the variance) under the assumptions of scheme 3, was introduced either in 1983, 1985, 1987 or 1989. The parameter set was as defined for simulation run number 2 in table 5.

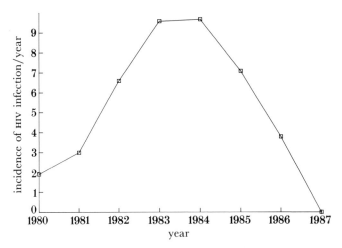

FIGURE 21. The observed change in the incidence of new HIV infections (recorded as a percentage of the cohort sample) in a group of male homosexuals in Amsterdam over the time period 1980–1987 (data from van Griesven et al. 1989).

this period, rather than as single-step change. In the absence of more detailed information we attempt to mimic a more continuous pattern of change by introducing two separate step changes in the mean rate of sexual partner change in the sexually active population and among new recruits to this population. These two changes (under the assumptions of scheme 3) are first from 8.7 to 5.0 per year and second from 5.0 to 3.35 per year. The simulated trajectories of the incidence of AIDS through time, for different times for the introductions of the two step changes in behaviour are recorded in figure 22. On the basis of the evidence recorded in the study of Evans *et al.* (1989) in London from 1984–1987, introducing the first step change in 1986 would appear to most closely mirror what actually happens in the U.K. Admittedly on the basis of limited information, we therefore tentatively suggest that the likely pattern of the epidemic in the male homosexual population in England and Wales may be similar to the lower

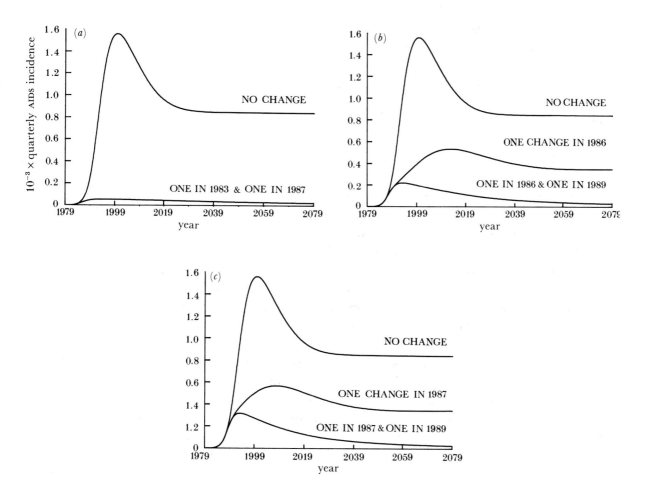

FIGURE 22. The influence of two consecutive reductions in sexual partner change rates on the quarter yearly incidence of AIDS. The parameter set used in the simulations was as defined for run number 2 in table 5 and the assumption concerning how the changes occurred and who they influence was as defined by scheme 3. In the different graphs, the two step changes were introduced at different time points. In (a) the changes occurred in 1983 and 1987, in (b) they occurred in 1986 and 1989, and in (c) they occurred in 1987 and 1989. The change introduced at the first time point was a reduction in the mean rate of partner change from 8.7 to 5.0 per year and that induced at the second time point was from 5.0 to 3.3 per year. For the purpose of comparison simulations under a one step change (from a mean rate of 8.7 per year to a mean of 5.0 per year) and no change at all (a mean of 8.7 per year throughout) are also recorded in graphs (a)–(c).

trajectories recorded in figure 22 b, c. In these simulations, the incidence of AIDS peaks at around 200–300 new cases per quarter year in 1989–1990 and thereafter slowly declines over a period of many decades.

5. DISCUSSION

Our numerical studies of the behaviour of a simple model of the transmission of HIV in a male homosexual population well illustrate the dangers inherent in making predictions about the future course of the AIDS epidemic in the U.K. Even simple models, based on the assumption of proportionate mixing, contain many parameters associated with the description of the incubation and infectious periods, and the distribution of rates of sexual partner change. Estimates of the values of these parameters are difficult to derive on the basis of published epidemiological research so far. Far too little attention has been devoted to the quantitative measurement and description of the parameters and processes that determine the overall pattern of the epidemic. This obviously needs to be rectified in future epidemiological research. However, even with the best intentions in mind many practical and ethical problems surround the measurement of many of the key parameters. As such, a marked improvement in the current state of affairs is unlikely to occur in the next few years. We are therefore left in the difficult position of trying to provide scientific information about future trends for health-care planning on a rather flimsy web of empirical data. On the basis of past trends in the rise in incidence of AIDS through time, plus limited data on the mean level of sexual activity within homosexual communities over the period 1979–1986, it seems likely that the average transmission probability $\bar{\beta}$ is of the order of 0.01. However, the relative durations (T_is) and intensities (β_is) of the two phases of infectiousness can have a marked impact on the course of epidemic even within the constraint of an average rate (β) of the magnitude of 0.01. If we assume that the first and last phases of infectiousness have durations of 1 and 3 years respectively (with a $\bar{\beta}$ of 0.01) then the model can provide a reasonable fit to observed trends even in the absence of any assumption concerning changes in sexual behaviour. A comparison of observation with model prediction is presented in figure 23 with the assumption that the yearly immigration rate of newly infected persons from Africa and the U.S.A. was of the order of 20 per year from 1979 to 1985 (we believe this to be a reasonable assumption on the basis of published data on risk factors associated with diagnosed cases of AIDS in the U.K. over this period). Aside from the uncertainties associated with the magnitude of the T_is and the β_is, future trends will be greatly influenced by the average incubation period of the disease. In the absence of nationwide serological data for the general population we are unable at present to check on our assumption of an eight-year average incubation period, by relating reported cases to the number of infected persons in the male homosexual population. Our estimate of the average period may well increase as data accumulates. Resolution of this problem would be greatly facilitated by good serological data derived from large-scale surveys (anonymous screening without consent).

Changes in sexual behaviour throughout the course of the epidemic further complicate the issue of predicting future trends. Changes have undoubtedly occurred but data are not available on their type and magnitude. The numerical studies of model behaviour under differing assumptions concerning the form and type of such changes clearly illustrate that a detailed knowledge of how such changes have taken place, and who has changed behaviour,

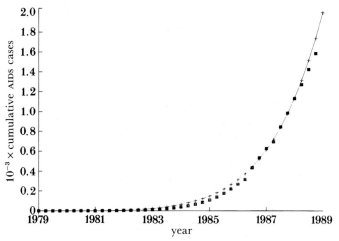

FIGURE 23. A comparison of the observed trend in reported AIDS cases in the U.K. among male homosexuals (recorded as cumulative cases) and the predictions of the model. (■) Data, (+) model. The epidemic was initiated in the model simulation in 1979 and the immigration rate of infected persons from outside the U.K. (i.e. from the U.S.A. or Africa) was set at 20 per year over the period 1979–1985. The parameter set employed was as defined for simulation run number 2 in table 5. Sexual behaviour was unchanged in the simulation in the period 1979–1989.

is essential for making projections into the future. At present the importance of recording summary statistics of the full distribution of rates of sexual partner change per unit of time is not widely appreciated by those concerned with research on sexual behaviour. For example a recent study by Fay *et al.* (1989), on patterns of sexual behaviour among male homosexual populations in the U.S.A. in 1979 and 1988 is excellent in the attention given to sampling method and data reliability. However, information on distributions of rates of sexual partner change per lifetime of same-gender sexual activity (clearly stratified by age and other factors) is not presented in a form that either records, or allows the calculation of summary statistics such as the mean or variance. This problem requires careful attention in future studies on sexual behaviour if our understanding of the transmission dynamics of HIV is to improve. The major issue illustrated by the numerical studies of simulated changes in sexual behaviour concerns the benefits to be gained from the induction of such changes early in the timecourse of the epidemic. This point is most clearly illustrated in figure 22. A simple comparison of the top and bottom trajectories of predicted cases of AIDS in graphs (a)–(c) reveals the enormous benefit that accrues from a reduction in the mean rate of sexual partner change (and an associated reduction in the variance) from around 8.7 to 3.3 per year in two steps early on in the protected timecourse. The induced reduction in the mean is of the order of 60% (from its pristine value) and yet this results in more than a 90% reduction in the cumulative number of AIDS cases over the 100-year timespan of the simulated epidemic. The moral is clear: resources used in education and publicity early on in the epidemic have a much greater impact in the long term, than resources used at a later stage. A second point of practical importance illustrated by the simulations concerns the question of who to target education at. The numerical studies reveal that the greatest immediate impact on the rate at which new cases of infection arise is achieved if reductions in the rate of sexual partner change occur in the infected subpopulation. In other words, education that aims to change behaviour must be directed not only at those who have not as yet joined the sexually active individuals who are still uninfected, but also, and most importantly, at those who are already infected (see figure 19).

One of the major objectives of the present study was to attempt to provide some general insights (both qualitative and quantitative) into the likely pattern of the epidemic in male homosexuals in the U.K. over the coming decades. We have stressed the difficulties inherent in attempting such projections, given the paucity of knowledge about key epidemiological parameters and processes. However, given the urgency of providing some guidelines, even if based on limited data, we draw attention to the projections recorded in figure 22. Under the crude assumption of a reduction in the mean rate of sexual partner change from 8.7 per year in 1985 to 5.0 per year in 1986 and to 3.35 per year in 1989 model projections suggest that the incidence of AIDS may plateau at around 200–300 cases per quarter year in 1989/90 and thereafter slowly decline over a period of many decades. The number of infected male homosexuals (HIV seropositive) in the U.K. at the period of peak incidence of disease is predicted to be somewhere between 10000–15000. If the average incubation period is significantly longer than eight years then the above figures will underestimate the true picture and we may expect a longer linear phase of the epidemic (reported cases of AIDS) over the coming five years.

The model employed in our numerical studies can be subject to various improvements and refinements. The major areas that require attention, aside from better parameter estimates, concern the assumption of proportionate mixing in sexual contacts and the need to introduce age structure to take account of changes in sexual activity with age. The question of 'who mixes with whom' with respect to individuals in different sexual activity classes is an important one. A number of recent studies have attempted to assess the impacts of different assumptions ranging from the extreme of virtually all contacts occurring within a given sexual activity class to the baseline assumption of proportionate mixing (Koopman et al. 1988; Hyman & Stanley 1988; May & Anderson 1989). Such studies are unfortunately rather abstract in character at the moment because of the absence of any data on the degrees of connectance within and between sexual activity classes. There is an urgent need for information in this area. The issue of age dependency is of obvious importance and this could be relatively easily incorporated within the structures of existing models. Limited data exist on patterns of change with age in the rate of acquiring new partners (see Fay et al. 1989; Anderson 1988 b). Fully age-structured models that allow varying degrees of mixing between and within different sexual activity classes will of course contain many more parameters for which estimates are required. An additional problem is the scale and cost of the numerical problems surrounding the investigation and analysis of the behaviours of such models.

In conclusion, we have restricted our attention to the spread of HIV among male homosexuals and tentatively suggested that changes in sexual behaviour may have resulted in the epidemic being close to, or at, its point of peak incidence (with respect to cases of AIDS) at present. This is encouraging but it should not be interpreted as implying that the problem is being conquered in the U.K. First, and foremost, the observed changes in behaviour among male homosexuals must be maintained in order to prevent a second upsurge in the incidence of new infections. Second, the virus is continuing to spread in other high-risk groups such as heterosexuals and intravenous drug users. A recent survey in London, for example, recorded a prevalence of HIV antibody of 1.6% in heterosexuals and 5.7% in intravenous drug users (Public Health

Laboratory Service Working Group 1989). A different study, also in London, recorded a rise in seroprevalence of HIV antibody in heterosexuals attending sexually transmitted disease clinics from 0.5% in January 1986 to 1.0% in 1987 (Loveday *et al.* 1989). These figures give cause for concern. Whether or not there will be a widely disseminated epidemic among heterosexuals in the U.K. remains uncertain. However, as we have noted elsewhere, if the case reproductive rate among heterosexuals is just above unity, the doubling time of the epidemic will be of the order of eight or more years (Anderson & May 1988). As such, in the first decade of its spread, changes in the general population from a fraction of 1% infected to some large fraction of 1% infected, will be extremely difficult to detect. Continued vigilance and increased efforts to improve epidemiological knowledge are clearly required under these circumstances.

R. M. Anderson and S. P. Blythe thankfully acknowledge financial support for this research from the Medical Research Council. We have all greatly benefited from discussions with Robert May, F.R.S.

Appendix A

At a non-trivial steady state we have:

$$0 = \Lambda(s) - (\lambda^* s + \mu)\, x^*(s), \tag{A 1}$$

$$\frac{\partial y^*(u, s)}{\partial u} = -(v(u) + \mu)\, y^*(u, s), \tag{A 2}$$

$$y^*(0, s) = \lambda^* s x^*(s), \tag{A 3}$$

with

$$\lambda^* = \frac{\displaystyle\int_0^\infty s' \int_0^\infty \beta(u)\, y^*(u, s)\, \mathrm{d}u\, \mathrm{d}s'}{\displaystyle s'\left[x^*(s) + \int_0^\infty y^*(u, s)\, \mathrm{d}u\right]\mathrm{d}s'}. \tag{A 4}$$

Writing

$$Y^*(s) = \int_0^\infty y^*(u, s)\, \mathrm{d}u, \tag{A 5}$$

then (A 2), (A 3) become

$$0 = \lambda^* s x^*(s) - \int_0^\infty v(u)\, y^*(u, s)\, \mathrm{d}u - \mu Y^*(s),$$

$$= \lambda^* s x^*(s)\, (1 - Q) - \mu Y^*(s) \tag{A 6}$$

(Blythe & Anderson 1988 *a*, *c*) where

$$Q = \int_0^\infty f(u)\, \mathrm{e}^{-\mu u}\, \mathrm{d}u, \tag{A 7}$$

and

$$f(u) = v(u) \exp\left\{-\int_0^u v(u'\, \mathrm{d}u')\right\}, \tag{A 8}$$

in the p.d.f. of the incubation period. Writing

$$B(s) = \lambda^* s x^*(s) L, \tag{A 9}$$

$$L = \int_0^\infty S(u)\, e^{-\mu u}\, du, \tag{A 10}$$

and

$$S(u) = \sum_{j=1}^N (\beta_j/\sigma_j) \sum_{i=1}^j b_{j,i}\, e^{-\sigma u}, \tag{A 11}$$

for $f(u)$ described by a series of N distinct exponential distributions with decay parameters $\{\sigma_j\}$, for each of which there is a fixed level of infectiousness $\{\beta_j\}$, with

$$b_{ji} = \prod_{k=1}^j \sigma_k \prod_{\substack{k=1 \\ k \ne i}}^i (\sigma_k - \sigma_j) \tag{A 12}$$

(details in Blythe & Anderson 1988b), (A 4) may now be written

$$\lambda^* = \frac{\displaystyle\int_0^\infty s'\beta(s')\, ds'}{\displaystyle\int_0^\infty s'[x(s') + Y^*(s')]\, ds'}, \tag{A 13}$$

which, using (A 6), becomes

$$\int_0^\infty s^* x^*(s)\, ds + \int_0^\infty s^2 x^*(s)\, ds \left[\frac{(1-Q)}{\mu}\lambda^* - L\right] = 0. \tag{A 14}$$

Hence defining

$$\hat{s} = \int_0^\infty s^2 x^*(s)\, ds \Big/ \int_0^\infty s x^*(s)\, ds \tag{A 15}$$

(see Blythe & Anderson 1988c), we have

$$\lambda^* = \frac{\mu}{1-Q}(L - 1/\hat{s}), \tag{A 16}$$

which provides condition

$$\rho = L\hat{s} > 1, \tag{A 17}$$

for endemic persistence of the infection.

For the multi-stage infection model (Blythe & Anderson 1988b), we have

$$L = \sum_{j=1}^N \frac{\beta}{\sigma_j} \sum_{i=1}^j \frac{b_{ji}}{\sigma_j + \mu}. \tag{A 18}$$

In the model and in this paper, $\beta_1 > 0$, $\beta_2 = 0$, $\beta_3 > 0$, $\sigma_1 \ne \sigma_2 \ne \sigma_3$ so (A 18) becomes,

$$L = \frac{\beta_1}{\sigma_1 + \mu} + \frac{\beta_3}{k_2}\frac{\sigma_1 \sigma_2 k_1}{k_3}, \tag{A 19}$$

where

$$k_1 = (\sigma_2 + \mu)(\sigma_3 + \mu)(\sigma_3 - \sigma_2) - (\sigma_1 + \mu)(\sigma_3 + \mu) + (\sigma_3 - \sigma_1) + (\sigma_1 + \mu)(\sigma_2 + \mu)(\sigma_2 - \sigma_1), \tag{A 20}$$

$$k_2 = (\sigma_1 + \mu)(\sigma_2 + \mu)(\sigma_3 + \mu), \tag{A 21}$$

$$k_3 = (\sigma_2 - \sigma_1)(\sigma_3 - \sigma_1)(\sigma_3 - \sigma_2). \tag{A 22}$$

Following Blythe & Anderson (1988c), we obtain values for λ^* and $\hat{s}$ by solving the equation

$$\int_0^\infty \frac{s\Lambda(s)}{s\lambda^*+\mu}\left\{1+s\left[\frac{(1-Q)}{\mu}\lambda^*-L\right]\right\}ds = 0, \tag{A 23}$$

for λ^*, and calculating

$$\hat{s} = \mu/[\mu L-(1-Q)\lambda^*]. \tag{A 24}$$

Defining X_i^* as the steady-state population size of the ith susceptible class, and

$$x_i^* = \int_{s_i}^{s_{i+1}} \frac{\Lambda(s)}{s\lambda^*+\mu}ds, \tag{A 25}$$

as the steady-state value for equivalent range of s in the continuum model, we may follow Blythe & Anderson (1988c) and define:

$$s_i = \frac{1}{\lambda^*}(\Lambda_i/x_i^*-\mu). \tag{A 26}$$

Then if the jth activity class has activity level c_j, and the rest have levels $c_i = s_i(i \neq j)$, then $c_j = s_j'$, any solution of

$$s' = \tfrac{1}{2}[\hat{s}+\lambda^*K \pm [(\hat{s}+\lambda^*K)^2+4\mu K]^{\frac{1}{2}}, \tag{A 27}$$

where

$$K = -\sum_{\substack{i=1\\i\neq j}}^{N} s_i(s_i-s)\,x_i^*. \tag{A 28}$$

Subject to the constrain $s_j \leqslant s_j' < s_{j+1}$.

The choice of the 'balancing class' j is arbitrary, but for $N = 6$ Blythe & Anderson (1988c) found $j = 5$ was an appropriate choice.

REFERENCES

Albert, J., Pehrson, P. O., Schulman, S., Hakansson, C., Lovhagen, G., Burgland, O., Beckman, S. & Funyo, E. M. 1988 HIV isolation and antigen detection in infected individuals and their seronegative sexual partners. *AIDS* 2, 107–112.

Allain, J. P. 1986 Prevalence of HTLV-III/LAV antibodies in patients with haemophilia and in their sexual partners in France. *New Engl. J. Med.* 315, 517.

Allain, J. P., Laurian, Y., Paul, D. A., Verroust, F. & Laurian, M.-J. 1987 Long term evaluation of HIV antigen and antibodies to p24 and gp41 in patients with haemophilia. *New Engl. J. Med.* 317(18), 1114–1121.

Anderson, R. M. 1988 The role of mathematical models in the study of HIV transmission and the epidemiology of AIDS. *J. AIDS* 1, 241–256.

Anderson, R. M. 1989 The epidemiology of H1V infection: variable incubation plus infectious periods and heterogeneity in sexual activity. *Jl R. statist. Soc.* A 151(1), 66–93.

Anderson, R. M. & Grenfell, B. T. 1986 Quantitative investigations of different vaccination policies for the control of congenital rubella syndrome (CRS) in the United Kingdom. *J. Hyg., Camb.* 96, 305–333.

Anderson, R. M. & Johnson, A. M. 1989 Rates of sexual partner change in homosexual and heterosexual populations in the United Kingdom. In *Kinsey Institute Conference on Sexual Behaviour in Relation to AIDS* (ed. B. Voller). New York: Oxford University Press. (In the press.)

Anderson, R. M. & May, R. M. 1984 Spatial, temporal and genetic heterogeneity in host populations and the design of immunization programmes. *IMA J. Math. appl. Med. Biol.* 1, 233–266.

Anderson, R. M. & May, R. M. 1986 The invasion, persistence and spread of infectious diseases within animal and plant communities. *Phil. Trans. R. Soc. Lond.* B 314, 533–570.

Anderson, R. M. & May, R. M. 1988 Epidemiological parameters of HIV transmission. *Nature, Lond.* 333, 514–519.

Anderson, R. M. & Medley, G. F. 1988 Epidemiology of HIV infection and AIDS: incubation and infectious periods, survival and vertical transmission. *AIDS* 2 (suppl.), S57–S64.

Anderson, R. M., Medley, G. F., Blythe, S. P. & Johnson, A. M. 1987 Is it possible to predict the minimum size of the acquired immunodeficiency syndrome (AIDS) epidemic in the United Kingdom? *Lancet* i, 1073–1076.

Anderson, R. M., Medley, G. F., May, R. M. & Johnson, A. M. 1987 A preliminary study of the transmission dynamics of the human immunodeficiency virus (HIV), the causative agent of AIDS. *IMA J. Math. appl. Med. Biol.* **3**, 229–263.

Antonen, J., Ranki, A., Valle, S.-L. & Krohn, K. 1988 A three-year immunological follow-up of HIV infected persons. Abstract number 4148. *IVth Int. Conf. AIDS, Stockholm.*

Antonen, J., Ranki, A., Valle, S., Seppala, E., Vapaatalo, H., Suni, J. & Krohn, K. 1989 The validity of immunological studies in HIV infection: a three year follow-up of 235 homo- or bisexual persons. *ACTA path. microbiol. Scand.* C **95**, 275–282.

Auerbach, D. M., Darrow, W. W., Jaffe, H. W. & Curran, J. W. 1989 Cluster of cases of AIDS. *Am. J. Med.* **76**, 487–500.

Auger, I., Thomas, P., De Gruttola, V., Morse, D., Moore, D., Williams, R., Truman, B. & Lawrence, C. E. 1988 Incubation periods for paediatric AIDS patients. *Nature, Lond.* **336**, 575–577.

Ayoola, E. A., Osisanya, J. O. S., Ukoli, P. *et al.* 1988 HIV-infections AIDS: Preliminary report on sero-prevalence and socio-cultural studies. In *XIIth International Congress for Tropical Medicine and Malaria, Abstracts* (ed. P. A. Kager & A. M. Polderman), p. 65. London: Elsevier Science.

Baldwin, J. D. & Baldwin, J. I. 1988 Factors affecting AIDS-related sexual risk-taking behaviour among college students. *J. Sex. Res.* **1**, 181–196.

Barbour, A. D. 1989 Macdonald's model and the transmission of bilharzia. *Trans. R. Soc. Trop. Med. Hyg.* **72**, 6–15.

Biggar, R., Goedert, J., Mann, D., Grossman, R., DiGioia, R., Sanchez, W., Melbye, M. & Blattner, W. 1988 Helper and suppressor lymphocyte changes in a cohort of homosexual men followed 5 years. Abstract number 4118. *IVth Int. Conf. AIDS, Stockholm.*

Biggar, R. J., Johnson, B. K., Oster, D., Sarlin, P. S., Ocheng, D., Tukei, P., Nsanze, H., Alexander, S., Bodner, A. J., Siongok, T. A., Gallo, R. C. & Blattner, W. A. 1985 Regional variation in prevalence of antibody against HTLV I and III in Kenya. *Int. J. Cancer* **35**, 763–767.

Blythe, S. P. & Anderson, R. M. 1988 Variable infectiousness in HIV transmission models. *IMA J. Math. appl. Med. Biol.* **5**, 181–200.

Blythe, S. P. & Anderson, R. M. 1988 Distributed incubation and infectious periods in models of the transmission dynamics of the Human Immunodeficiency Virus (HIV). *IMA J. Math. appl. Med. Biol.* **5**, 1–19.

Blythe, S. P. & Anderson, R. M. 1988 Heterogeneous sexual activity models of HIV transmission in male homosexual populations. *IMA J. Math. appl. Med. Biol.* **5**, 237–260.

Blythe, S. P. & Anderson, R. M. 1989 Modelling changes in sexual behaviour in HIV transmission models with heterogeneous sexual activity and variable infectiousness. *IMA J. Math. appl. Med. Biol.* **5**, 237–260.

Blythe, S. P. & Castillo-Chavez, C. 1989 Like-with-like preference and sexual mixing models. (In preparation.)

BMRB 1989 *AIDS advertising campaign: report for surveys during the first year of advertising.* London: British Market Research Board.

CDC 1987 Self-reported changes in sexual behaviors among homosexual and bisexual men from the San Francisco City Clinic Cohort. *Morbid. Mortal. wkly Rep.* **36**, 187–189.

CDC 1988 *A review of current knowledge and plans for expansion of HIV surveillance activities.* Washington: Department of Health and Human Services, Public Health Service and Centres for Disease Control.

CDC 1989 Acquired immunodeficiency syndrome in the San Francisco cohort study. 1978–1985. *Morbid. Mortal. wkly Rep.* **38**, 573–575.

Carne, C. A., Johnson, A. M., Pearce, F., Smith, A., Tedder, R. S., Weller, I. V. D., Loveday, C., Hawkins, A., Williams, P. & Adler, M. W. 1987 Prevalence of antibodies to human immunodeficiency virus, gonorrhoea rates, changed sexual behaviour in homosexual men in London. *Lancet* i, 656–658.

Carne, C. A., Weller, I. V. D., Loveday, C. & Adler, M. W. 1987 From PGL to AIDS: who will progress? *Br. Med. J.* **294**, 868–869.

Carne, C. A., Weller, W. D., Sutherland, S. *et al.* 1985 Rising prevalence of human T-lymphotropic virus type III (HTLV III) infection in homosexual men in London. *Lancet* i, 1261–1262.

Castello-Branco, L., Carvalho, M. I. L., de Castilho, E. A., Pereira, H. E., Pereira, M. S. & Galvao-Castro, B. 1988 Frequency of antibody to human immunodeficiency virus (HIV) in male and female prostitutes in Rio de Janeiro, Brazil. Abstract number 5144. *IVth Int. Conf. AIDS, Stockholm.*

Castillo-Chavez, C., Hethcote, H. W., Andreasen, V., Levin, S. A. & Liu, W.-M. 1988 Cross-immunity in the dynamics of homogeneous and heterogeneous populations. In *Mathematical Ecology* (ed. T. G. Hallam, L. G. Gross & S. A. Levin), pp. 303–316. Singapore: World Scientific Publishing Co.

Castillo-Chavez, C., Hethcote, H. W., Andreasen, V., Levin, S. A. & Liu, W.-M. 1989 Epidemiological models with age structure, proportionate mixing, and cross-immunity. *J. Math. Biol.* (In the press.)

Chikwem, J. O., Ola, T. O., Gashau, W., Chikwem, S. D., Bajami, M. & Mambula, S. 1988 Impact of health education on prostitutes' awareness and attitudes to AIDS. *Publ. Hlth, Lond.* **102**, 439–445.

Coates, R. A., Read, S., Fanning, M., Shepherd, F., Calzavara, L., Johnson, K., Soskolne, C. & Klein, M. 1988 Transmission of HIV in male sexual contacts of men with ARC or AIDS. Abstract number 4113. *IVth Int. Conf. AIDS, Stockholm.*

Cohen, J. E. 1987 Sexual behaviour and randomized responses. *Science, Wash.* **236**, 1503.

Cooper, L. N. 1986 Theory of an immune system retrovirus. *Proc. natn. Acad. Sci. U.S.A.* **83**, 9159–9163.

Cornet, P., Laga, M., Bonneux, L., Piot, P. & Taelman, H. 1988 Case control study of risk factors for HIV infection among African adults residing in Belgium. *IVth Int. Conf. AIDS, Stockholm*. (In the press.)

Costa, M. F. F. L., Oliveira, M. R., Oliveira, E. I., Paulino, U. H. M., Guimaraes, M. D. C., Munoz, A., Proietti, F. A., Antunes, C. M. F. & Greco, D. B. 1988 Risk factors for AIDS or AIDS-related complex among homo/bisexual men in Minas Gerais, Brazil. *IVth Int. Conf. AIDS, Stockholm*. (In the press.)

Costagliola, D., Brouard, N., Mary, J. & Valleron, A. J. 1988 Incubation time for AIDS: implications of different probability distribution models. Abstract number 4698. *IVth Int. Conf. AIDS, Stockholm*.

Coutinho, R. A., Goudsmit, J., Paul, D. A. *et al.* 1987 The natural history of HIV infection in homosexual men. In *Acquired Immunodeficiency Syndrome* (ed. J. C. Gluckman & E. Vilmer). New York: J. Wiley.

Coutinho, R. A., Schoonhoven, F. J., van den Hoek, J. A. R. & Emsbroek, J. A. 1987 Influence of special surveillance programmes and AIDS on declining incidence of syphilis in Amsterdam. *Genitourin. Med.* **63**, 210–213.

Cox, D. R. & Medley, G. F. 1989 A process of events with notification delay and the forecasting of AIDS. *Phil. Trans. R. Soc. Lond.* B **325**, 135–145. (This volume.)

Crovari, P., Penco, G., Valente, A., Imberciadori, G., Di Ponzio, A., Calderisis, S., Angeli, C. & Cuneo-Crovari, P. 1988 HIV infection in two cohorts of drug addicts prospectively studied. Association of serological markers with clinical progression. Abstract number 4527. *IVth Int. Conf. AIDS, Stockholm*.

Curran, J. W., Jaffe, H. W., Hardy, A. M., Meade Morgan, W. M., Selik, R. M. & Dondero, T. J. 1988 Epidemiology of HIV infection and AIDS in the United States. *Science, Wash.* **239**, 610–616.

Curran, J. W., Meade Morgan, W., Hardy, A. M., Jaffe, H. W., Darrow, W. W. & Dowdle, W. R. 1985 The epidemiology of AIDS: current status and future prospects. *Science, Wash.* **229**, 1352–1357.

De Vincenzi, I. 1988 Heterosexual transmission of HIV: a European community multicentre study. *IVth Int. Conf. AIDS, Stockholm*.

de Wolf, F., Lange, J., Houweling, J., Coutinho, R., Schellekens, P. T., van der Noordaa, J. & Goudsmit, J. 1988 Numbers of CD4+ cells and levels of core antigen of the antibodies to HIV as predictors of AIDS among seropositive homosexual men. *J. infect. Dis.* **158**(3), 615–622.

de Wolf, F., Lange, J., Schellekens, P., Coutinho, R., van der Noordaa, J. & Goudsmit, J. 1988 Natural history of HIV infection in homosexual males monitored by immunological and virological parameters. *IVth Int. Conf. AIDS, Stockholm*. (In the press.)

Des Jarlais, D. C., Friedman, S. R., Marmor, M., Cohen, H., Mildvan, D., Yancovitz, S., Mathur, U., El Sadr, W., Spira, T. J., Garber, J., Beatrice, S. T., Abdul-Quader, A. S. & Sotheran, J. L. 1987 Development of AIDS, HIV seroconversion, and potential cofactors for T4 cell loss in a cohort of IV drug users. *AIDS* **1**, 105–111.

Detels, R., Visscher, B. R., Fahey, J. L., Sever, J. L., Gravell, M., Madden, D. L., Schwartz, K., Dudley, J. P., English, P. A., Power, H., Clark, V. A. & Gottlieb, M. S. 1987 Predictors of clinical AIDS in young homosexual men in a high risk area. *Int. Epid. Assoc.* 271–276.

Dietz, K. & Hadeler, K. P. 1988 Epidemiological models for sexually transmitted diseases. *J. Math. Biol.* **26**, 1–25.

Dietz, K. & Schenzle, D. 1985 Proportionate mixing models for age-dependent infection transmission. *J. Math. Biol.* **22**, 117–120.

Edison, R., Feigal, D. W., Kirn, D. & Abrams, D. A. 1988 Progression of laboratory values, AIDS morbidity, and mortality in 6-year cohort with PGL. Abstract number 4145. *IVth Int. Conf. AIDS, Stockholm*.

El Sadr, W., Marmor, M., Zolla-Pazner, S., Stahl, R. E., Lyden, M., William, D., D'Onofrio, S., Weiss, S. H. & Saxinger, C. 1987 Four year prospective study of homosexual men. *J. infect. Dis.* **155**(4), 789–793.

Elmslie, K., Romanowski, B., Hankins, C., Rekart, M., Hammond, G., Fralick, R., Millson, E., Gemmill, I. & O'Shaughnessy, M. 1988 Canadian collaborative study of women attending Sexually Transmitted Diseases (STD) Clinics. Abstract number 4064. *IVth Int. Conf. AIDS, Stockholm*.

European Collaborative Group 1988 Mother-to-Child Transmission of HIV Infection. *Lancet* ii, 1039–1042.

Evans, B. A., McLean, K. A., Dawson, S. G., Teece, S. A., Bond, R. A., MacRae, K. D. & Thorp, R. W. 1989 Trends in sexual behaviour and risk factors for HIV infection among homosexual men, 1984–87. *Br. med. J.* **298**, 215–218.

Eyster, M. E., Gail, M. H., Ballard, J. O., Al-Mondhiry, H. & Goedert, J. J. 1987 Natural history of HIV infection in haemophiliacs: effects of T cell subsets, platelet counts, and age. *Ann. int. Med.* **107**(i), 1–6.

Ezzell, C. 1988 Tests for new AIDS treatment being in three clinics. *Nature, Lond.* **334**, 557.

Fay, R. E., Turner, C. F., Klassen, A. D. & Gagnon, J. H. 1989 Prevalence and patterns of same-gender sexual contact among men. *Science, Wash.* **243**, 338–348.

Fischl, M., Fayne, T., Flanagan, S., Ledan, M., Stevens, R., Fletcher, M., LaVoie, L. & Trapido, E. 1988 Seroprevalence and risks of HIV infections in spouses of persons infected with HIV. Abstract reference number 4060. *IVth Int. Conf. AIDS, Stockholm*.

Fischl, M., Trapido, E., Stevens, R., Fayne, T., Flanagan, S., Resnick, L. & LaVoie, L. 1988 Seroprevalence of HIV antibody in a sexually active heterosexual population. *IVth Int. Conf. AIDS, Stockholm*. (In the press.)

Fischl, M. A., Dickinson, G. M., Scott, G. B., Klimas, N., Fletcher, M. A. & Parks, W. 1987 Evaluation of heterosexual partners, children, and household contacts of adults with AIDS. *J.A.M.A.* **257**, 640–644.

Fox, R., Odaka, N. J., Brookmeyer, R. & Polk, B. F. 1987 Effects of HIV antibody disclosure on subsequent sexual activity in homosexual men. *AIDS* i, 241–245.

Garcia, S., de la Loma, A. & Romero, J. 1988 Non blood heterosexual transmission of HIV infection. Abstract number 4003. *IVth Int. Conf. AIDS, Stockholm.*

Gellan, M. C. A. & Ison, C. A. 1986 Declining incidence of gonorrhoea in London. A response to fear of AIDS. *Lancet* ii, 920.

Georgoulias, V., Fountouli, D., Karvela-agelakis, A., Komios, G., Malliarakis-pinetidous, E., Antoniados, G., Samakidis, K., Kondakis, X., Papapetropoulou, M., Zoumbos, N., Axenidou, O., Makris, K. & Sonidis, G. 1988 HIV1 and HIV2 in Greece. *Annls int. Med.* **108**(1), 155.

Gerstoft, J., Petersen, C. S., Kroon, S., Ullman, S., Lindhardt, B. O., Hofman, B., Gaub, J. & Dickmeiss, E. 1987 The immunological and clinical outcome of HIV infection: 31 months of follow-up in a cohort of homosexual men. *Scan. J. inf. Dis.* **19**, 503–509.

Ginzberg, H. M., Fleming, P. L. & Miller, K. D. 1988 Selected public health observations derived from the MACS. *J. AIDS* **1**, 2–7.

Ginzburg, H. M., Fleming, P. L. & Miller, K. D. 1988 Selected public health observations derived from the multicenter AIDS cohort study. *J. AIDS* **1**, 2–8.

Goedert, J. J., Biggar, R. J., Melbye, M., Mann, D. J., Wilson, S., Gail, M. H., Grossman, R. J., Digiola, R. A., Sanchez, W. C., Stanley, H., Weiss, S. H. & Blattner, W. A. 1987 Effect of T4 count and cofactors on the incidence of AIDS in homosexual men infected with HIV. *J. Am. med. Ass.* **257**(3), 331–334.

Goedert, J. J., Biggar, R. J., Weiss, S. H., Eyster, E. M., Melbye, M., Wilson, S., Ginzburg, H. M., Grossman, R. J., Digioia, R. A., Spira, T. J., Giron, J. A., Ebbesen, P., Gallo, R. C. & Blattner, W. A. 1986 Three year incidence of AIDS in five cohorts of HTLV III-Infected Risk Group Members. *Science, Wash.* **231**, 992–995.

Goedert, J. J., Eyster, M. E., Biggar, R. J. & Blattner, W. A. 1987 Heterosexual transmission of HIV. *AIDS Res. & Hum. Retro.* **3**(4), 355–361.

Goedert, J. J., Eyster, M. E., Ragni, M. V., Biggar, R. J. & Gail, M. H. 1988 Rate of heterosexual HIV transmission and associated risk with HIV-antigen. Abstract 4019. *IVth Int. Conf. AIDS, Stockholm.*

Goilav, C., Prinsen, H. & Piot, P. 1988 Incidence of HIV infection and sexual practices in gay men in a low endemic area. *IVth Int. Conf. AIDS, Stockholm.* (In the press.)

Gottlieb, M. S., Detels, R. & Fahey, J. L. 1987 T-cell phenotyping in the diagnosis and management of AIDS and AIDS-related disease. *Annls Inst. Pasteur/immunol.* **138**, 135–143.

Goudsmit, J., Wolf, F., Paul, D. A. *et al.* 1986 Expression of human immunodeficiency virus antigens (HIV-Ag) in serum and cerebrospinal fluid during acute and chronic infection. *Lancet* ii, 177–180.

Grant, R. M., Wiley, J. A. & Winkelstein, W. 1987 Infectivity of the Human Immunodeficiency Virus: estimates from a prospective study of homosexual men. *J. infect. Dis.* **156**, 189–193.

Greenblatt, R. M., Lukehart, S. A., Plummer, F. A., Quinn, T. C., Critchlow, C. W., Ashley, R. L., D'Costa, L. J., Ndinya-achola, J. O., Corey, L., Ronald, A. R. & Holmes, K. K. 1988 Genital ulceration as a risk factor for HIV infection. *AIDS* **2**, 47–50.

Griensven, G. J. P., Vroome, E. M. M., Goudsmit, J. & Coutinho, R. A. 1989 Changes in sexual behaviour and the fall in incidence of HIV infection among homosexual men. *Br. med. J.* **298**, 218–221.

Groopman, J. E., Caiazzo, T., Thomas, M. A., Ferriani, R. A., Saltzman, S., Moon, M., Seage, G., Horsburgh, R. C. & Mayer, K. 1988 Lack of evidence of prolonged HIV infection before antibody seroconversion. *Blood* **71**(6), 1752–1754.

Guydish, J. & Coates, T. 1988 Changes in AIDS-related high risk behaviour among heterosexual men. Abstract number 4072. *IVth Int. Conf. AIDS, Stockholm.* (In the press.)

Hanraham, J. P., Wormser, G. P., Reilly, A. A., Maguire, B. H., Gavis, G. & Morse, D. L. 1984 Prolonged incubation period of AIDS in intravenous drug abuse: epidemiological evidence in prison inmates. *J. infect. Dis.* **150**, 263–266.

Harrer, T., Meyer, E. & Kalden, J. R. 1988 Follow-up of HIV-infected homosexuals with lymphadenopathy syndrome (LAS). Abstract number 4102. *IVth Int. Conf. AIDS, Stockholm.*

Haseltine, W. A. & Sodroski, J. G. 1987 *Annls Inst. Pasteur/virol* 83–92.

Haseltine, W. A. & Sodroski, J. G. 1987 Cell membrane fusion mediated by the envelope glycoproteins on the primary effector of AIDS virus cytopathicity. *Annls Inst. Pasteur/immunol* **138**, 83–92.

Hessol, N. A., Lifson, A. R., Rutherford, G. W., O'Malley, P. M., Franks, D. R., Darrow, W. W. & Jaffe, H. W. 1988 Cofactors for progression of HIV infection in a cohort of homosexual and bisexual men: a decade of epidemiologic research. *IVth Int. Conf. AIDS, Stockholm.*

Hessol, N. A., Rutherford, G. W., Lifson, A. R., O'Malley, P. M., Doll, L. S., Darrow, W. W., Jaffe, H. W. & Werdegar, D. 1988 The natural history of HIV infection in a cohort of homosexual and bisexual men: A decade of follow-up. *IVth Int. Conf. AIDS, Stockholm.*

Hethcote, H. W. & Van Ark, J. W. 1987 Epidemiological models for heterogeneous populations: proportionate mixing, parameter estimation and immunization programs. *Math. Biosci.* **84**, 85–118.

Hethcote, H. W. & Yorke, J. A. 1984 Gonorrhoea transmission dynamics and control. In *Lecture Notes in Biomathematics No. 56*. New York: Springer-Verlag.

Hira, S., Wadhawan, D., Nkowane, B., Kamanga, J. & Perine, P. 1988 Heterosexual transmission of HIV in Zambia. Abstract number 4006. *IVth Int. Conf. AIDS, Stockholm.*

HMSO 1988 *Short-term prediction of HIV infection and AIDS in England and Wales.* London: Her Majesty's Stationery Office.

Hudson, C. P., Hennis, A. J. M., Kataaha, P., Lloyd, G., Moore, A. T., Sutehall, G. M., Whetstone, R., Wreghitt, T. & Karpas, A. 1988 Risk factors for the spread of AIDS in rural Africa. *AIDS* 2, 255–260.

Hyman, J. M. & Stanley, E. A. 1988 Using mathematical models to understand the AIDS epidemic. *Math. Biosci.* 90, 415–474.

Iwasa, Y., Andreasen, V. & Levin, S. 1987 Aggregation in model ecosystems, I, perfect aggregation. *Ecol. Monogr.* 37, 287–302.

Jacquez, J. A., Simon, C. P. & Koopman, K. 1988 Modelling and analysing HIV transmission: the effect of contact patterns. *Math. Biosci.* 92, 119–199.

Jaffe, H., Choi, K., Thomas, P. A., Haverkos, H. W., Auerbach, D. M., Guinan, M. E., Rogers, M. F., Spira, T. J., Darrow, W. W., Kramer, M. A., Friedman, S., Monroe, J. M., Friedman-kien, A. E., Laubenstein, L. J., Marmor, M., Safai, B., Dritz, S. K., Crispi, S. J., Fannin, S. L., Orkwis, J. P., Kelter, A., Rushing, W. R., Thacker, S. B. & Curran, J. W. 1983 National case control study of KS and PCP in homosexual men. *Annls int. Med.* 99(2), 145–159.

Jama, J., Grillner, L., Biberfeld, G., Osman, S., Isse, A., Abdirahman, M. & Bygdeman, S. 1987 Sexually transmitted viral infections in various population groups in Mogadishu, Somalia. *Genitourin. Med.* 63, 329–332.

Jason, J., Lui, K., Ragni, M., Darrow, W. & Hessol, N. 1988 Risk of developing AIDS in HIV-infected cohorts of haemophilic and homosexual men. Abstract number 4139. *IVth Int. Conf. AIDS, Stockholm.*

Jason, J. M., McDougal, J. S., Dixon, G., Lawrence, D. N., Kennedy, M. S., Hilgartner, M., Aledort, L. & Evatt, B. L. 1986 HTLV-III/LAV antibody and immune status of household contacts and sexual partners of persons with haemophilia. *J. Am. med. Ass.* 255, 212–215.

Johnson, A. M. & Gill, O. N. 1989 Evidence for recent changes in sexual behaviour in homosexual men in England and Wales. *Phil. Trans. R. Soc. Lond.* B 325, 153–161. (This volume.)

Johnson, A. M., Petherick, A., Davidson, S., Howard, L., Osborne, L., Sonnex, C., Robertson, R., Tchamouroff, S., Hooker, M., McLean, K., Brettle, R. & Adler, M. W. 1988 Transmission of HIV to heterosexual partner of infected men and women. *IVth Int. Conf. AIDS, Stockholm.*

Jones, P., Hamilton, P. J., Bird, G., Fearns, M., Oxley, A., Tedder, R., Cheingsong-Popov, R. & Codd, A. 1985 AIDS and haemophilia: morbidity and mortality in a well defined population. *Br. med. J.* 291, 695–699.

Kalbfleish, J. A. & Lawless, J. F. 1988 Estimating the incubation period for AIDS patients. *Nature, Lond.* 333, 504–505.

Kamradt, T., Niese, D. & Kamps, B. 1988 Incubation period of AIDS in haemophiliacs. *Nature, Lond.* 333, 402.

Kamradt, T. G. A., Niese, D., Schneweis, K. E., Brackmann, H. H. & Kamps, B. S. 1988 Heterosexual transmission of HIV in haemophiliacs. Abstract number 4008. *IVth Int. Conf. AIDS, Stockholm.*

Kaplan, J. E., Spira, T., Fishbein, D. & Pinsky, P. 1988 Natural history of HIV infection in homosexual men with lymphadenopathy syndrome; relationship with T-helper cell count. *IVth Int. Conf. AIDS, Stockholm.*

Kaplan, J. E., Spira, T., Fishbein, D. & Pinsky, P. 1988 Evidence for increasing risk of developing AIDS in men with HIV-associated lymphadenopathy syndrome. A 6-year follow-up. *IVth Int. Conf. AIDS, Stockholm.*

Karlsson, A., Morfeldt-Mansson, L., Bottiger, B., Bratt, G., Furucrona, A., Bottiger, M., Sandstrom, E. *et al.* 1988 The Venhalsan, Stockholm cohort after 4.4 years a clinical and immunological update. *IVth Int. Conf. AIDS, Stockholm.*

Kingsley, L. A., Kaslow, R., Rinaldo, C. R., Detre, K., Odako, N., van Raden, M., Detels, R., Polk, B. F., Chmiel, J., Kelsey, S. F., Ostrow, D. & Visscher, B. 1987 Risk factors for seroconversion to human immunodeficiency virus among male homosexuals. *Lancet* i, 345–348.

Konings, E., Anderson, R. M., Morley, D., O'Riordan, T. & Meegan, M. 1989 Rates of sexual partner change among two pastoralist nilotic groups in East Africa. *AIDS* 3, 245–247.

Koopman, J., Simon, C. & Jacquez, J. 1988 Sexual partner selectiveness: Effects on homosexual HIV transmission dynamics. *J. AIDS* 1, 486–504.

Kreiss, J. K., Kitchen, L. W., Prince, H. E., Kasper, C. K. & Essex, M. 1985 Antibody to HTLV III in wives of haemophiliacs. *Annls Int. Med.* 102, 623–626.

Kreiss, J. K., Koech, D., Plummer, F. A., Holmes, K. K., Lightfoote, M., Piot, P., Ronald, A. R., Ndinya-achola, J. O., D'Costa, L. J., Roberts, P., Ngugi, E. N. & Quinn, T. C. 1986 AIDS virus infection in Nairobi prostitutes. *New Engl. J. Med.* 314(7), 414–418.

Laga, M., Taelman, H., Bonneux, L., Cornet, P., Vercauteren, G. & Piot, P. 1988 Risk factors for HIV infection in heterosexual partner of HIV infected Africans and Europeans. Abstract number 4004. *IVth Int. Conf. AIDS, Stockholm.*

Laurian, Y., Peynet, J. & Verroust, F. 1989 HIV infection in sexual partners of HIV seropositive patients with haemophilia. *New Engl. J. Med.* 320, 183.

Lawrence, C., Thomas, P., Morse, D., Truman, B., Auger, I., Williams, R. & DeGruttola, V. 1988 Incubation periods for maternally transmitted pediatric AIDS cases. Abstract number 7268. *IVth Int. Conf. AIDS, Stockholm.*

Lawrence, D. N., Jason, J. M., Holman, R. C., Evatt, B. L., Starcher, E. T. *et al.* 1988 Heterosexual transmission of HIV in female partners of HIV-infected U.S. haemophilic men. Abstract number 4009. *IVth Int. Conf. AIDS, Stockholm.*

Loveday, C., Pomeroy, L., Weller, I. V. D., Quirk, J., Hawkins, A., Williams, H., Smith, A., Williams, P., Tedder, R. S. & Adler, M. W. 1989 Human immunodeficiency viruses in patients attending a sexually transmitted disease clinic in London, 1982–1987. *Br. med. J.* **298**, 419–422.

Lui, K.-J., Darrow, W. W. & Rutherford, G. W. 1988 A model based estimate of the mean incubation period for AIDS in homosexual men. *Science, Wash.* **240**, 1333–1339.

Lui, K., Lawrence, D. N., Morgan, W. M., Peterman, T. A., Haverkos, H. W. & Bregman, D. J. 1986 A model-based approach for estimating the mean incubation period of transfusion-associated acquired immuno-deficiency syndrome. *Proc. natn. Acad. Sci. U.S.A.* **83**, 3051–3055.

Mann, J. M., Nzilambi, N., Piot, P., Bosenge, N., Kalala, M., Francis, H., Colebunders, R. C., Azila, P. K., Curran, J. W. & Quinn, T. C. 1988 HIV infection and associated risk factors in female prostitutes in Kinshasa, Zaire. *AIDS* **2**, 249–254.

Maw, R. D., Connolly, J., Johnston, S., Mckirgan, J., McNeill, J. & Russell, J. 1987 Follow up study of STD sexual practice and HIV serology in homosexual men attending an STD clinic. *Genitourin. Med.* **63**, 279–280.

May, R. M. & Anderson, R. M. 1987 Transmission dynamics of HIV infection. *Nature, Lond.* **326**, 137–142.

May, R. M. & Anderson, R. M. 1988 The transmission dynamics of the human immunodeficiency virus (HIV). *Phil. Trans. R. Soc. Lond.* B **321**, 565–607.

May, R. M. & Anderson, R. M. 1989 Heterogeneities, cofactors, and other aspects of the transmission dynamics of HIV/AIDS. *Current Topics in AIDS.* (In the press.)

McEvoy, M. & Tillet, H. E. 1985 Some problems in the prediction of future numbers of cases of the acquired immunodeficiency syndrome in the U.K. *Lancet* ii, 541–542.

McKusick, L., Horstman, W. & Coates, T. J. 1989 AIDS and sexual behaviour reported by gay men in San Francisco. *Am. J. publ. Hlth* **75**, 493–496.

McKusick, L., Wiley, J. A., Coates, T. J. & Stall, G. 1985 Reported changes in the sexual behaviour of men at risk from AIDS, San Francisco 1982–84: the AIDS Behavioural Research Project. *Publ. Hlth Rep.* **100**, 622–629.

Medley, G. F., Anderson, R. M., Cox, D. R. & Billard, L. 1987 Incubation period of AIDS in patients infected via blood transfusion. *Nature, Lond.* **328**, 719–721.

Medley, G. F., Anderson, R. M., Cox, D. R. & Billard, L. 1988 Estimating the incubation period for AIDS patients. *Nature, Lond.* **333**, 504–505.

Medley, G. F., Billard, L., Cox, D. R. & Anderson, R. M. 1988 The distribution of the incubation period for the Acquired Immunodeficiency Syndrome (AIDS). *Proc. R. Soc. Lond.* B **233**, 367.

Miller, E. T., Miller, K. K., Goldman, E., Griffiths, P. D. & Kernoff, P. B. A. 1987 Low risk of anti HIV seroconversion in female sexual partners of haemophiliacs and their children. *III Int. Conf. AIDS, Washington.*

Mohammed, I., Chikwem, J. O. & Williams, E. E. 1988 Prevalence of Human Immunodeficiency Virus Type 1 (HIV 1) infection among female prostitutes in two Nigerian states. Abstract number 5143. *IVth Int. Conf. AIDS, Stockholm.* (In the press.)

Moss, A. R., Bacchetti, P., Osmond, D., Krampf, W., Chaisson, R. E., Stites, D., Wilber, J., Allain, J. P. & Carlson, J. 1988 Seropositivity for HIV and the development of AIDS or ARC: three year follow-up of San Francisco General Hospital cohort. *Br. med. J.* **296**, 745–750.

Moss, A. R., Osmond, D., Bacchetti, P., Chaisson, R., Krampf, W. & Ross, E. 1988 Predicting progression to AIDS: implication of the San Francisco General Hospital Cohort Study for early intervention. Abstract number 4137. *IVth Int. Conf. AIDS, Stockholm.*

Nold, A. 1980 Heterogeneity in disease transmission modelling. *Math. Biosci.* **52**, 227–240.

Norman, C. 1985 AIDS trends: projections from limited data. *Science, Wash.* **230**, 1020–1021.

Nzila, Nzilambi, Ryder, R., Colebunders, R., Ndilu, M., LeBughe, M., Kamenga, M., Kashamuka, M., Brown, C. & Francis, H. 1988 Married couples in Zaire with discordant HIV serology. Abstract number 4059. *IVth Int. Conf. AIDS, Stockholm.* (In the press.)

Padian, N., Glass, S., Marquis, L., Wilney, J. & Winkelstein, W. 1988 Heterosexual transmission of HIV in California: results from a heterosexual partner's study. Abstract number 4020. *IVth Int. Conf. AIDS, Stockholm.*

Padian, N., Marquis, L., Francis, D. P., Anderson, R. E., Rutherford, G. W., O'Malley, P. & Winkelstein, W. 1987 Male to female transmission of HIV. *J. Am. med. Ass.* **258**(6), 788–790.

Pederson, C., Nielsen, C., Vestergaard, B. F., Gerstoff, J., Krogsgaard, K. & Nielsen, J. E. 1987 Temporal relation of antigenaemia and loss of antibodies to core antigens to development of clinical disease in HIV infection. *Br. med. J.* **295**, 567–569.

Peterman, T. A. & Curran, J. W. 1986 Sexual transmission of HIV. *J. Am. med. Ass.* **256**(16), 2222–2226.

Peterman, T. A., Stoneburner, R. L., Allen, J. R., Jaffe, H. W. & Curran, J. W. 1988 Risk of HIV transmission from heterosexual adults with transfusion associated interactions. *J. Am. med. Ass.* **259**(1), 55–59.

Piot, P., Plummer, F. A., Rey, M., Ngugi, E. N., Rouzious, C., Ndinya-achola, J. O., Nsanze, H., Veracauteren, G., D'Costa, L. J., Laga, M., Fransen, L., Haase, D., van der Groen, G., Brunham, R. C., Ronald, A. R. & Brun-Vezinet, F. 1987 Retrospective and seroepidemiology of AIDS virus infection in Nairobi populations. *J. infect. Dis.* **155**(6), 1108–1112.

Piot, P., Taelman, H., Minlangu, K. B., Mbendi, N., Ndangi, K., Kalambayi, K., Bridts, C., Quinn, T. C., Feinsod, F. M., Wobin, O., Mazebo, P., Stevens, W., Mitchell, S. & McCormick, J. B. 1984 AIDS in a heterosexual population in Zaire. *Lancet* ii, 65–69.

Plummer, F. A., Ngugi, E. N., Simonsen, J. N., Cameron, D. W., Bosire, M., Waiyaki, P., Ronald, A. R. & Ndinya-achola, J. O. 1988 Prevention of HIV transmission through health education and promotion of condoms among high risk prostitutes. (In preparation.)

Plummer, F. A., Simonsen, J. N., Cameron, D. W., Ndinya-achola, J. O., Kreiss, J. K., Gakinya, M., Waiyaki, P., Karasira, P., Cheang, M., Piot, P., Ronald, A. R., Bosire, M., Kimata, J., D'Costa, L. J. & Ngugi, E. N. 1989 Co-factors in male to female sexual transmission of HIV. *Int. J. Epidemiol.* (In the press.)

Public Health Laboratory Service Working Group 1989 Prevalence of HIV antibody in high and low risk groups in England. *Br. med. J.* **298**, 422–423.

Quinn, T. C., Glasser, D., Cannon, R. O., Matuszak, D. L., Dunning, R. W., Kline, R. L., Campbell, C. H., Israel, E. M., Fauci, A. M. & Hook, E. W. 1988 HIV infection among patients attending clinics for sexually transmitted diseases. *New Engl. J. Med.* **318**(4), 197–203.

Rees, M. 1987 The sombre view of AIDS. *Nature, Lond.* **326**, 343–345.

Rees, M. 1988 AIDS incubation period in haemophiliacs. *Nature, Lond.* **332**, 312.

Rogers, M., Starcher, T., Bush, T. & Ward, J. 1988 Epidemiology of pediatric transfusion-acquired AIDS (T-A AIDS) in the United States. Abstract number 4586. *IVth Int. Conf. AIDS, Stockholm.*

Rogers, M. F., Thomas, P. A., Starcher, E. T., Noa, M. C., Bush, T. J. & Jaffe, H. W. 1987 AIDS in children: report of the CDC national surveillance 1982–1985. *Pediat.* **79**(6), 1008–1014.

Sattenspiel, L. 1987 Population structure and the spread of disease. *Hum. Biol.* **59**, 411–438.

Sattenspiel, L. 1987 Epidemics in non-randomly mixing populations: a simulation. *Am. J. Phys. Anthrop.* **73**, 251–265.

Sattenspiel, L. & Simon, C. P. 1989 The spread and persistence of infectious diseases in structural populations. *Math. Biosci.* (In the press.)

Schechter, M. T., Craib, K. J. P., Willoughby, B., Sestak, P., Weaver, M. S., Douglas, B. *et al.* 1988 Progression to AIDS in a cohort of homosexual men: results at 5 years. Abstract number 4098. *IVth Int. Conf. AIDS, Stockholm.*

Schwartlader, B. 1988 A prospective multicenter cohort study in homosexual men in the FRG. Abstract number 4101. *IVth Int. Conf. AIDS, Stockholm.*

Scott, G. B., Fischl, M. A., Klimas, N., Fletcher, M. A., Dickinson, G. D., Levine, R. S. & Parks, W. P. 1985 Mothers of infants with AIDS. *J. Am. med. Ass.* **253**(3), 263–266.

Seildain, M., Krasinski, K., Bebenroth, D., Itri, V., Paolino, A. M. & Valentine, F. 1988 Prevalence of HIV infection in New York call girls. *J. AIDS* **1**, 150–154.

Selwyn, P. A., Shoenbaum, E. E., Hartel, D., Klein, R. S., Davenny, K., Friedland, G. H. *et al.* 1988 AIDS and HIV-related mortality in intravenous drug users. Abstract number 4526. *IVth Int. Conf. AIDS, Stockholm.*

Sewankambo, N. K., Carswell, J. W., Mugerwa, R. D., Lloyd, G., Kataaha, P., Downing, R. G. & Lucas, S. 1987 HIV infection through normal heterosexual contact in Uganda. *AIDS* **1**, 113–116.

Simmonds, P., Lainson, F. A. L., Cuthbert, R., Steel, C. M., Peutherer, J. F. & Ludham, C. A. 1988 HIV antigen and antibody detection: variable responses to infection in the Edinburgh haemophiliac cohort. *Br. med. J.* **296**, 593–598.

Stanley, E. A. 1989 Mathematical models of the AIDS epidemic: an historical perspective. 'Lectures in Complexity' Santa Fe Institute Studies in the Science of Complexity, Reading, M.A., Vol. III. (In preparation.)

Staszewski, S., Rehmet, S., Hofmeister, W. D., Helm, E. B., Stille, W., Werner, A. & Doerr, H. W. 1988 Analysis of transmission rates in heterosexually transmitted HIV infection. Abstract reference 4068. *IVth Int. Conf. AIDS, Stockholm.*

Steigbigel, N. H., Maude, D. W., Feiner, C. J., Harris, C. A., Saltzman, B. R., Klein, R. S. *et al.* 1988 Heterosexual transmission of HIV infection. *IVth Int. Conf. AIDS, Stockholm.*

Steizbigel, N. H., Maude, D. W., Feiner, C. J., Harris, C. A., Saltzman, B. R., Klein, R. S. *et al.* 1987 Heterosexual transmission of infection of disease by the HIV. *III Int. Conf. AIDS, Washington.*

Taelman, H., Bonneux, L., Cornet, P., van der Groen, G. & Piot, P. 1987 Transmission of HIV to partners of seropositive heterosexuals from Africa. *III Int. Conf. AIDS, Washington.*

Tirelli, U., Vaccher, E., Saracchini, S., Errante, D., Bullian, P. L. & Zagonel, V. 1988 Detection of HIV infection in male prostitutes. *IVth Int. Conf. AIDS, Stockholm.* (In the press.)

Titti, F., Verani, P., Butto, S., Reza, G., Ippolito, G., Perucci, C., Rapicetta, M. & Rossi, G. B. 1988 Seroepidemiology of HIV in a cohort of Italian homosexual men. Abstract number 4104. *IVth Int. Conf. AIDS, Stockholm.*

Vaccher, E., Saracchini, S., Errante, D., Bullian, P., Zappala, E., Pinna, C., Serraino, D., Martelli, P. & Tirelli, U. 1988 Progression of HIV disease among intravenous drug abusers (IVDA): A three year prospective study. Abstract number 4529. *IVth Int. Conf. AIDS, Stockholm.*

van de Perre, P., Carael, M., Robert-Guroff, M., Gallo, R. C., Clumeck, N., Nzabinhimana, E., De Mol, P., Butzler, J.-P. & Kanyamupira, J.-B. 1985 Female prostitutes, a risk group for infection with human T-cell lymphotropic virus type III. *Lancet* ii, 524–527.

van den Hoek, J. A. R., van Ilaastrecht, H. J. A., Scheeringa-Troost, B., Goudsmit, J. & Coutinho, R. A. 1988 HIV-infection and sexually transmitted diseases (STD) among addicted prostitutes in Amsterdam; the potential of HIV-transmission. *IVth Int. Conf. AIDS, Stockholm.* (In the press.)

Webber, J. N., Rogers, L. A., Scott, K., Bernie, C., Harris, J. R. W., Wadsworth, J., Moshtael, O., McManus, T., Jeffries, D. J. & Pinching, A. J. 1986 Three year prospective study of HTLV-III/LAV infection in homosexual men. *Lancet* i, 1179–1182.

Weller, I. V. D. 1986 The AIDS virus: a new human immunodeficiency retrovirus and the natural history of infection. *J. Hepatol.* 1, 127–138, Appendix 13.

Weller, I. V. D., Hindley, D. J., Adler, M. W. & Melchum, J. T. 1984 Gonorrhoea in homosexual men and media coverage of the acquired immune deficiency syndrome, 1982–3. *Br. med. J.* 289, 1041–1042.

Winkelstein, W., Lyman, D. M., Padian, N., Grant, R., Samuel, M., Wiley, J. A., Anderson, R. E., Lang, W., Riggs, J. & Levy, J. A. 1987 Sexual practices and risk of infection by the human immunodeficiency virus: The San Francisco Men's Health Study. *J. Am. med. Ass.* 257, 321–325.

Winkelstein, W., Samuel, M., Padian, N. S., Wiley, J. A., Lang, W., Anderson, R. M. & Levy, J. A. 1987 The San Francisco Men's Health Study: III. Reduction in Human Immunodeficiency Virus transmission among homosexual/bisexual men, 1982–86. *Am. J. Publ. Hlth* 76, 685–689.

Winkelstein, W., Wiley, J. A., Padian, N. & Levy, J. A. 1986 Potential for transmission of AIDS associated retrovirus from bisexual men in San Francisco to their female sexual contacts. *J. Am. med. Ass.* 255(7), 901–902.

Zulaica, D., Arrizabalaga, J., Iribarren, J. A., Perez-Trallero, E., Rodriguez-Arrondo, F. & Garde, C. 1988 Follow-up of 100 HIV infected intravenous drug abusers. Abstract no. 3018, *IVth Int. Conf. AIDS, Stockholm.*

Phil. Trans. R. Soc. Lond. B **325**, 99–112 (1989)   [99]

Printed in Great Britain

POPULATION PROJECTIONS FOR AIDS USING AN ACTUARIAL MODEL

By A. D. WILKIE

R. Watson & Sons, Consulting Actuaries, Watson House, London Road, Reigate RH2 9PQ, U.K.

This paper gives details of a model for forecasting AIDS, developed for actuarial purposes, but used also for population projections. The model is only appropriate for homosexual transmission, but it is age-specific, and it allows variation in the transition intensities by age, duration in certain states and calendar year.

The differential equations controlling transitions between states are defined, the method of numerical solution is outlined, and the parameters used in five different Bases of projection are given in detail. Numerical results for the population of England and Wales are shown.

1. INTRODUCTION

This paper describes a model for forecasting AIDS, which was designed originally for actuarial use in dealing with life assurance companies and pension funds, but which is also applicable to making projections for AIDS in a total population.

The mathematical model was first outlined in Wilkie (1988 *a*), and described more fully in Wilkie (1988 *b, c*). Since those papers were written, certain enhancements have been made that are described in this paper.

Population projections for the United Kingdom have appeared in Wilkie (1987), Daykin (1987 *a*), Cox, Working Group Report (1988) and Daykin *et al.* (1988). Results applicable to life assurance and Permanent Health Insurance have appeared in Daykin (1987 *b*, 1988) and Daykin *et al.* (1988). Some revised projections, using some of the enhancements referred to above, have appeared in Daykin (1989).

In Appendix 10 of Cox, Working Group Report (1988) forecasts were given for the population of England and Wales up to 1992. Here, we extend the results up to the year 2012. It is not suggested that these forecasts, on any of the bases used, can be reliable for such a long period ahead, but they show the results of the model for such longer periods; these may be of assistance in understanding the consequences of particular assumptions.

Actuaries require that the model should be age-specific, and should take into account normal age-specific mortality as well as the extra sickness and mortality from AIDS. In this respect this model is more elaborate than most others that have been proposed, though it is less elaborate in other directions.

Any practical model must simplify the complexity of the real world. This actuarial model simplifies the reality of AIDS by assuming that the only mode of transmission of HIV infection is through sexual activity among male homosexuals, and that all reported cases in the United Kingdom have been among homosexuals. This simplification appears reasonable because 84 % of reported cases in the U.K. have been among homosexuals. However, it ignores the separate transmission dynamics among haemophiliacs, drug users and heterosexual males and females that in due course may come to play a larger part in the total epidemic of HIV infection.

A further simplification is the assumption that all those males described below as being 'at risk' of infection behave in the same manner at any one time, so that the chance of infection depends on the age of the individual at risk and the particular calendar year, but not on any subcategorization according to frequency of sexual contact or frequency of change of sexual partner.

The model treats males of any single age as forming a 'cohort', and tracks their experience independently of any other cohort. The assumption that only those of the same age infect one another is artificial, but, if infections between those of different ages balance out, it can be considered to be an adequate representation of the truth.

2. THE MODEL

The members of one cohort at age x may be in any one of the eleven discrete states that are indicated in figure 1. Five of these are live states: 'clear', 'at risk', 'immune', 'positive' and 'sick from AIDS'. Six are dead states; these are kept separate simply to show the live state that someone died in. The dead states are: 'dead from clear', 'dead from at risk', 'dead from immune', 'dead from positive', 'dead from sick (other than from AIDS)' and 'dead from AIDS'. It may not be possible to distinguish the last two categories, but calculated deaths other than from AIDS of those who suffer from AIDS are comparatively trivial.

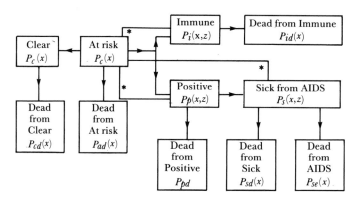

Figure 1 : AIDS Model : States and Transitions
(*denotes possible infection)

Those in the clear state are those whose assumed sexual activity is such that they run no risk whatever of becoming infected with HIV. They form the 'normal' pre-AIDS population for comparative purposes. Those in the at risk state are treated as exposing themselves to the risk of acquiring HIV infection by reason of sexual contact with infected people. Those in the immune state are assumed to have acquired HIV infection and to be infectious, but to be wholly immune from becoming sick from AIDS or dying from AIDS. Whether such a state can exist is not known, but its existence has been suggested by Anderson *et al.* (1986), and it is not difficult to implement this feature of the model.

Those in the positive state are HIV seropositive, but not yet sick from AIDS; they are infectious and not immune. It is assumed that it is possible to distinguish between those who are HIV seropositive and those who are sick from AIDS in a discrete way. In reality there are several stages in the transition from HIV infection to death from AIDS. Those who are suffering from AIDS are thought to be highly infectious, but it is possible that their sexual activity may be considerably reduced. The model makes it possible to choose whether those sick from AIDS are treated as contributing to further infections or not.

It is assumed that the current age (x) is part of the total status, and that transition intensities can all vary by current age. In addition, since each age cohort (or year of birth cohort) is treated separately, each transition intensity can also be varied by calendar year, so that each cohort has its own set of transition intensities.

Duration since entry to the states immune, positive and sick from AIDS are also relevant to the transition intensities. This duration is denoted in each case as z.

Conditional on some initial distribution at a starting age x_0, the probability of an individual being in state j (or the proportion of individuals in state j) at age x is denoted by $p_j(x)$, where $j = [c, a, cd, ad, id, pd, sd, se \text{ (dead from AIDS)}]$, as in figure 1. The corresponding density for those in the immune, positive or sick from AIDS states at age x and duration z is $p_i(x, z)$, $p_p(x, z)$ or $p_s(x, z)$ respectively, and the total probability of being immune, positive or sick at all durations is denoted $p_i(x)$, $p_p(x)$ or $p_s(x)$.

Possible transitions are as shown in figure 1. Those in any of the live states may die, and those who are sick from AIDS may die from AIDS or from causes other than AIDS. Those who are at risk may change their behaviour and become clear, for example, by giving up sexual activity altogether, or by restricting themselves to one equally monogamous partner. There is no representation in the model of transfer from clear to at risk. Those who are at risk may become infected, and at that point are immediately allocated either to the immune state or to the positive state, in proportions that may depend on age (and on calendar year, though it seems unlikely that this would actually exercise any influence).

Those in the positive state may become sick from AIDS, if they do not die first. Infection is possible from the immunes, positives and sick to the at risk, and how this is represented is described below.

The transition intensity from state j to state k is generally represented by $\mu_{jk}(x)$, if it depends only on age, x, and by $\mu_{jk}(x, z)$ if it depends on both age, x, and duration, z.

3. DIFFERENTIAL EQUATIONS

The usual Kolmogorov differential equations describe the transitions between states, with the exception of the transmission of infection. The differential equations are now described.

$$\mathrm{d}p_c(x)/\mathrm{d}x = -\mu_{cd}(x)\,p_c(x) + \mu_{ac}(x)\,p_a(x); \tag{1}$$

clears are diminished by death and increased by transfers from at risk to clear.

$$\mathrm{d}p_a(x)/\mathrm{d}x = -\mu_{ac}(x)\,p_a(x) - \mu_{ad}(x)\,p_a(x) - T(x); \tag{2}$$

at risk are diminished by transfers to clear and to dead and by the term $T(x)$, representing transfers to the infectious states. This will be described below.

$$\mathrm{d}p_{cd}(x)/\mathrm{d}x = +\mu_{cd}(x)\,p_c(x); \tag{3}$$

dead from clear are increased by deaths among clears. Similar formulae apply to all the dead states.

Put $w = x - z$, so w is the entry age to the given state. Then, for $z > 0$,

$$\mathrm{d}p_i(w+z, z)/\mathrm{d}z = -\mu_{id}(x, z)\, p_i(x, z);$$ (4)

immunes at duration z are diminished only by death.

$$\mathrm{d}p_p(w+z, z)/\mathrm{d}z = -\mu_{pd}(x, z)\, p_p(x, z) - \mu_{ps}(x, z)\, p_p(x, z);$$ (5)

positives at duration z are diminished by death and by transfers to sick from AIDS.

$$\mathrm{d}p_s(w+z, z)/\mathrm{d}z = -\mu_{sd}(x, z) \cdot p_s(x, z) - \mu_{se}(x, z) \cdot p_s(x, z);$$ (6)

those sick from AIDS at duration z may die from causes other than AIDS or may die from AIDS. The new sick at duration 0 are given by,

$$\frac{\partial p_s(x, 0)}{\partial x} = \int_0^\infty \mu_{ps}(x, z)\, p_p(x, z)\, \mathrm{d}z.$$ (7)

New immunes at duration 0 are given by,

$$\partial p_i(x, 0)/\partial x = f_i(x)\, T(x),$$ (8)

where $f_i(x)$ is the proportion of those newly infected at age x who are assumed to enter the immune state, and $T(x)$ is the density of newly infected at age x.

New positives at duration 0 are given by

$$\partial p_p(x, 0)/\partial x = [1 - f_i(x)]\, T(x),$$ (9)

i.e. all those newly infected who do not enter the immune state.

To explain $T(x)$, the newly infecteds, we define terms relating to the total proportions immune, positive and sick at age x as

$$P_i(x) = \int_0^\infty k_i(x, z)\, p_i(x, z)\, \mathrm{d}z,$$ (10)

$$P_p(x) = \int_0^\infty k_p(x, z)\, p_p(x, z)\, \mathrm{d}z,$$ (11)

and

$$P_s(x) = \int_0^\infty k_s(x, z)\, p_s(x, z)\, \mathrm{d}z.$$ (12)

We also define;

$$A_i(x) = \int_0^\infty \mu_{ai}(x, z)\, p_i(x, z)\, \mathrm{d}z,$$ (13)

$$A_p(x) = \int_0^\infty \mu_{ap}(x, z)\, p_p(x, z)\, \mathrm{d}z,$$ (14)

and

$$A_s(x) = \int_0^\infty \mu_{as}(x, z)\, p_s(x, z)\, \mathrm{d}z.$$ (15)

Then

$$T(x) = p_a(x) \left(\frac{A_i(x) + A_p(x) + A_s(x)}{p_a(x) + P_i(x) + P_p(x) + P_s(x)} \right).$$ (16)

The intensities of infectivity, $\mu_{ai}(x, z)$, $\mu_{ap}(x, z)$ and $\mu_{as}(x, z)$, are a combination of what other authors have treated as two elements: frequency of sexual contact with a new partner, and probability of infection from a new partner. It is assumed that these intensities may vary by the age of the at risks, perhaps representing varying levels of sexual activity at different ages, and may also vary according to how long the partner has been infected.

The terms $k_i(x, z)$, $k_p(x, z)$ and $k_s(x, z)$ allow for the frequency with which immunes, positive and sick respectively enter the pool of sexual exchanges, relative to those at risk who are assumed to enter with unit relative frequency.

If there were no immunes or sick, if the infectivity intensity were a constant μ for all ages and durations, and if $k_p(x, z) = 1$, then the density of new infections would be

$$T(x) = p_a(x) \left(\frac{\mu p_p(x)}{p_a(x) + p_p(x)} \right), \tag{17}$$

which in the absence of any other transitions would lead to the usual logistic growth of the infected proportion in a population.

4. Numerical solution

The technique used is one developed by Waters & Wilkie (1987) that was originally designed to describe sickness with recovery for the purposes of Permanent Health Insurance.

A set of initial conditions is given, and discrete approximations to the differential equations are used to carry forward the initial conditions in steps of length h, where h is some convenient fraction of a year, usually one quarter.

Where duration enters into the status, it is also subdivided into steps of h, i.e. $(0, h)$, $(h, 2h)$, etc. The proportions positive, immune or sick with AIDS in each duration step are separately recorded and carried forward from step to step by a discrete approximation. The integrals that appear in equations (10) to (15) are approximated by summations.

Once the initial conditions in a particular starting year and the values of the transition intensities for each future year have been chosen, the forecast is wholly determined.

The model allows a very flexible representation of the transition intensities, varying by age, calendar year and where relevant also by duration in the current state. Our knowledge is too small at this stage to take full advantage of this flexibility.

5. Bases

For the forecasts shown in Appendix 10 of Cox, Working Group Report (1988) five different bases were used, denoted A, B, C, D and E. Although A in general produces the highest and E the lowest numbers, they should not be taken as representing upper and lower limits for the possible course of HIV infection in England and Wales. The reality may turn out to be different from any of these forecasts.

Although the possibility of representing an immune state exists in the model, it was not used in any of the five bases described. Those sick with AIDS were assumed not to contribute to new infections, so that infection was only possible from the positives, who contribute to the denominator of equation (16) to the same extent as the at risk, i.e. $k_p(x, z)$ was taken as unity for all x and z and $k_s(x, z)$ was taken as zero.

The five bases have many assumptions in common and these are described first; the differences are described later.

5.1. *Base Date*

Each projection commences at the end of 1983, and projects forward at annual intervals.

5.2. *Initial Population*

All five start with the estimated population of males aged 15–70 in England and Wales as at mid-1983 taken from 'Population Projections 1983–2023' (Office of Population Censuses and Surveys series PP2 No. 13; HMSO 1985), treated as if this population applied at the end of 1983.

5.3. *New Entrants*

All Bases assume that in each future year the number of males entering the 'population' at age 15 each year is the same as that projected in 'Population Projections 1983–2023'.

5.4. *Mortality other than from AIDS*

All Bases assume that the mortality other than from AIDS of those in the clear, at risk, positive and sick from AIDS statuses is the same as that experienced by the England and Wales male population in 1983, graduated according to the formula,

$$\mu_{ca}(x) = a_0 + a_1 t + \exp[b_0 + b_1 t + b_2(2t^2 - 1)], \tag{19}$$

where $t = (x - 70)/50$, a convenient transformation of age; $a_0 = -0.000\,780$; $a_1 = -0.001\,446$; $b_0 = -3.735\,111$; $b_1 = 4.725\,108$; $b_2 = -0.662\,952$. This was derived by graduating the available data using the methods described by Forfar *et al.* (1988).

5.5. *Intensity of developing AIDS (incubation rate)*

All Bases assume that the intensity of developing AIDS is given by a Gompertz formula $(\exp(-8.4 + 1.4d))$ with a maximum of 0.25, where d is the duration in years since infection.

TABLE 1. PERCENTAGE OF HIV POSITIVE DEVELOPING AIDS AFTER DURATION SHOWN ACCORDING TO FORMULA SHOWN IN TEXT

duration/years	modified Gompertz	Weibull
1	0.05	0.60
2	0.25	3.08
3	1.05	7.90
4	4.24	15.06
5	16.14	24.26
6	34.69	34.89
7	49.13	46.18
8	60.39	57.33
9	69.15	67.62
10	75.97	76.53
11	81.29	83.78
12	85.43	89.33
13	88.65	93.33
14	91.16	96.05
15	93.16	97.78
16	94.64	98.82
17	95.82	99.41
18	96.75	99.72
19	97.47	99.88
20	98.03	99.95

The proportion who have developed AIDS by the given number of years since HIV infection under this assumption are shown in table 1 and can be compared with those from a Weibull distribution with intensity $0.0143\,d^{1.383}$, which are also shown.

5.6. *Initial proportions positive*

For each Basis a particular proportion HIV-positive at each age is assumed in order that approximately the following number of new cases of AIDS in the years 1984 to 1987 are reproduced. In 1984 there were 109 new cases; 224 in 1985; 425 in 1986 and 762 in 1987. In each case it is assumed that there were no sick from AIDS at the end of 1983.

6. BASIS A

The assumptions used for basis A are listed below.

6.1. *Initial proportion not clear*

It is assumed that in 1983, 5% of the male population aged 21 to 50 were either at risk or positive. The proportion reduces linearly to 2% at age 15 and to zero at age 70. It is assumed that 2% of new entrants at age 15 in future years are at risk, and that a small fraction of these are positive.

6.2. *Transfer from at risk to clear*

It is assumed that there is no transfer from at risk to clear.

6.3. *Infection intensity*

It is assumed that this has a constant value of 0.7 from ages 25 to 35, reducing linearly outside this range to zero at ages 15 and 70. An infection intensity of 0.7 corresponds to a 'doubling time', in the initial stages of the epidemic, of approximately one year.

6.4. *Mortality of those sick from AIDS*

It is assumed that this is a constant rate of 0.7; this is equivalent to one half of those becoming sick from AIDS dying within one year, one half of the survivors dying within a second year and so on proportionately, giving an average survival time of 1.4 years.

7. BASIS B

The assumptions used for basis B are listed below.

7.1. *Initial proportion not clear*

The same as in basis A.

7.2. *Transfer from at risk to clear*

It is assumed that there is a constant transfer from at risk to clear at the rate of 0.1 per year from the beginning of 1987 onwards. This is equivalent to the numbers at risk reducing by 40% every five years in the absence of any other transitions.

7.3. *Infection intensity*

The pattern by age is the same as in basis A, and the rate to the beginning of 1987 is the same, but it is assumed that over the five years from the beginning of 1987 to 1992 the peak infection intensity of 0.7 reduces to 0.35, equivalent to the 'doubling time' itself doubling to two years over this period, and remaining constant thereafter.

7.4. *Mortality of those sick from* AIDS

The same as in basis A.

It can be seen that basis B assumes considerable changes in behaviour as compared with basis A in two ways: first a substantial proportion of those at risk change their behaviour entirely to join the clear status, and those who remain at risk reduce their rate of sexual activity or rate of change of sexual partners to one half of its previous level over the five years from 1987 to 1992. Alternatively this is compatible with an assumption that sexual behaviour is heterogeneous, and those with the highest rate of sexual activity become infected first, with the disease spreading later to those who have a lower rate of sexual activity. However, the model does not specifically represent this pattern.

8. BASIS C

The assumptions used for basis C are listed below.

8.1. *Initial proportion not clear*

Half the rates of bases A and B, i.e. 2.5% from ages 21–50, reducing to 1% at age 15 and to zero at age 70; new entrants in future years: 1%.

8.2. *Transfer from at risk to clear*

The same as in basis B.

8.3. *Infection intensity*

The same as in basis B.

8.4. *Mortality of those sick from* AIDS

The same constant rate as in basis A of 0.7 up to the beginning of 1987, reducing linearly over the five years to the beginning of 1992 to a level of 0.35. This represents a lengthening of the survival time of those sick with AIDS resulting from the use of drugs or other treatment. After 1992 the survival rate is such that 30% of those becoming sick with AIDS die within one year, 30% of the survivors within a second year and so on, giving an average survival time of 2.8 years.

Basis C makes the same assumptions as basis B about behavioural changes, and in addition assumes half the starting proportions to be not clear, and that Zidovudine (AZT) or other drugs have a significant effect in prolonging the life of those sick with AIDS. It is therefore a fairly 'optimistic' projection, whereas basis A assumes almost no change from the position in the early years (with the exception that those at younger ages and among future new entrants have a lower proportion not clear, i.e. behavioural change comes about in future cohorts rather than among present cohorts).

9. Basis D

The assumptions used for basis D are the same as those for basis B with two exceptions. The transfer from at risk to clear at a rate of 0.1 per year commences at the beginning of 1984, rather than at the beginning of 1987; and the reduction in the infection intensity takes place over the two years from the beginning of 1984 to the beginning of 1986, rather than from 1987 to 1992.

10. Basis E

The assumptions used for basis E are the same as those used for basis C, with the same two exceptions as differentiate basis D from basis B, that the transfer from at risk to clear commences at the beginning of 1984, not 1987, and that the reduction in infection intensity occurs over the two years from 1984 to 1986.

It can be seen that bases B, C, D and E form a sort of square table of bases, differentiated in pairs.

	5% at risk no AZT	2½% at risk AZT
behavioural change 1987–92	B	C
behavioural change 1984–86	D	E

11. Results

The results from the projections are shown in tables 2 to 7. The tables show: table 2, projected numbers of deaths from AIDS during each year from 1984 to 2012; table 3, projected numbers of new cases of AIDS during each year from 1984 to 2012; table 4, projected numbers of new HIV infections during each year from 1984 to 2012; table 5, projected numbers of persons currently sick from AIDS at the end of each year from 1983 to 2012; table 6, projected numbers HIV positive, but not sick from AIDS, at the end of each year from 1983 to 2012; table 7, projected total numbers of deaths from AIDS by the end of each year from 1983 to 2012.

It can be seen that basis A (in which no behavioural changes are assumed) produces greater numbers than any of the others. Basis B generally produces greater numbers in the early years than the remaining bases, except that, since those sick from AIDS live much longer in basis C than in basis B, there are more people sick from AIDS at any one time in basis C.

By the end of the century, however, basis D shows a greater number of new HIV infections than basis B, and in due course this would result in a greater number of new cases of AIDS and of deaths from AIDS in basis D than in basis B beyond the final date shown. The reason for this is that a reduction in the infection intensity, which occurs sooner in basis D than in basis B, postpones but does not necessarily eliminate new infections. If the conditions of equation (17) were maintained, then the available population would be 'saturated' in due course, whatever the value of the transition intensity, m. In the full model those in the at risk group who do not change their behaviour to become clear may become infected in the period before they get older when the transition intensities are assumed to reduce to zero. Similarly, basis C produces higher numbers than basis E until about the end of the century.

It is unrealistic to assume that the epidemic of HIV infection will continue with no change whatever in sexual behaviour, so the results from basis A should be taken as indicating a likely upper limit (subject to all the other assumptions being valid). The other bases are more realistic, but there is a very big difference between them. The peak year for numbers of new

TABLE 2. ENGLAND AND WALES MALE POPULATION: PROJECTED NUMBERS OF DEATHS FROM
AIDS DURING GIVEN YEAR

basis... year	A	B	C	D	E
1984	28	28	28	28	28
1985	96	96	96	96	96
1986	208	208	208	206	206
1987	415	415	394	403	383
1988	790	789	693	735	649
1989	1423	1419	1145	1200	985
1990	2477	2452	1784	1726	1310
1991	4241	4131	2635	2266	1571
1992	7078	6642	3986	2854	1942
1993	11305	9881	5905	3536	2490
1994	16961	13393	7864	4322	3059
1995	23545	16520	9535	5191	3630
1996	30035	18693	10680	6099	4170
1997	35282	19724	11234	6982	4640
1998	38518	19799	11277	7765	5003
1999	39557	19161	10926	8373	5234
2000	38678	18010	10294	8750	5320
2001	36391	16522	9479	8865	5266
2002	33253	14852	8566	8724	5089
2003	29760	13126	7618	8357	4812
2004	26293	11434	6686	7814	4464
2005	23092	9841	5802	7152	4072
2006	20267	8386	4990	6427	3662
2007	17835	7090	4259	5686	3254
2008	15762	5960	3616	4969	2863
2009	14002	4991	3059	4301	2500
2010	12506	4174	2582	3700	2173
2011	11239	3494	2179	3173	1882
2012	10172	2933	1842	2719	1630

TABLE 3. ENGLAND AND WALES MALE POPULATION: PROJECTED NUMBERS OF NEW CASES OF
AIDS DURING GIVEN YEAR

basis... year	A	B	C	D	E
1984	110	110	110	110	110
1985	216	216	216	215	215
1986	422	422	421	414	413
1987	811	811	806	771	769
1988	1490	1487	1465	1322	1312
1989	2577	2561	2474	1933	1901
1990	4417	4338	4064	2498	2422
1991	7454	7122	6380	3067	2917
1992	12097	10851	9152	3770	3490
1993	18462	14897	11668	4606	4117
1994	25979	18365	13283	5536	4736
1995	33292	20492	13741	6502	5279
1996	38830	21071	13223	7430	5685
1997	41662	20562	12174	8233	5908
1998	41796	19471	10941	8825	5932
1999	39849	17972	9643	9144	5768
2000	36595	16223	8362	9167	5449
2001	32721	14374	7156	8911	5019
2002	28757	12541	6060	8424	4524
2003	25066	10803	5090	7770	4006
2004	21838	9208	4249	7017	3495
2005	19114	7782	3534	6226	3016
2006	16840	6535	2934	5446	2582
2007	14932	5464	2438	4711	2200
2008	13318	4560	2032	4045	1873
2009	11943	3808	1702	3459	1597
2010	10772	3188	1435	2955	1368
2011	9783	2682	1220	2529	1179
2012	8962	2270	1048	2174	1025

TABLE 4. ENGLAND AND WALES MALE POPULATION: PROJECTED NUMBERS OF NEW HIV INFECTIONS DURING GIVEN YEAR

basis... year	A	B	C	D	E
1984	4795	4795	4696	4012	3933
1985	8546	8546	8136	4360	4186
1986	14890	14890	13469	4692	4388
1987	24778	23080	19164	5948	5372
1988	38079	29707	21794	7308	6292
1989	52018	32456	20677	8661	7005
1990	61355	30283	16896	9891	7407
1991	62311	24706	12371	10862	7441
1992	55962	20040	9217	11413	7099
1993	46257	17025	7324	11429	6455
1994	36452	13951	5691	10902	5625
1995	28058	11169	4373	9936	4734
1996	21486	8823	3349	8698	3876
1997	16750	6919	2572	7361	3109
1998	13694	5402	1987	6065	2461
1999	11920	4208	1552	4898	1936
2000	10864	3285	1234	3904	1528
2001	10078	2587	1007	3095	1221
2002	9356	2070	846	2462	997
2003	8651	1696	732	1985	838
2004	7985	1429	650	1637	726
2005	7397	1236	588	1388	647
2006	6921	1094	541	1209	588
2007	6574	987	505	1079	544
2008	6363	906	477	982	509
2009	6272	844	457	908	483
2010	6263	797	442	851	462
2011	6291	763	431	806	447
2012	6323	739	425	773	437

TABLE 5. ENGLAND AND WALES MALE POPULATION: PROJECTED NUMBERS SICK FROM AIDS AT END OF GIVEN YEAR

basis... year	A	B	C	D	E
1983	0	0	0	0	0
1984	82	82	82	82	82
1985	202	202	201	201	200
1986	414	414	413	407	407
1987	808	808	823	774	791
1988	1505	1503	1591	1358	1450
1989	2652	2638	2913	2085	2359
1990	4581	4512	5180	2848	3461
1991	7775	7484	8902	3638	4791
1992	12764	11664	14029	4539	6318
1993	19870	16635	19734	5589	7918
1994	28811	21544	25072	6779	9561
1995	38444	25433	29172	8062	11166
1996	47082	27710	31587	9358	12629
1997	53259	28433	32380	10568	13835
1998	56290	27978	31883	11578	14693
1999	56296	26654	30427	12293	15148
2000	53897	24728	28315	12647	15189
2001	49890	22438	25810	12624	14849
2002	45044	19986	23123	12250	14187
2003	39995	17525	20417	11587	13280
2004	35191	15167	17809	10712	12210
2005	30873	12983	15378	9708	11053
2006	27122	11014	13171	8650	9874
2007	23915	9281	11208	7601	8726
2008	21189	7783	9494	6607	7646
2009	18874	6511	8020	5698	6658
2010	16909	5446	6767	4891	5774
2011	15247	4563	5714	4191	4999
2012	13856	3839	4837	3595	4329

TABLE 6. ENGLAND AND WALES MALE POPULATION: PROJECTED NUMBER HIV+ (NOT SICK) AT
END OF GIVEN YEAR

basis... year	A	B	C	D	E
1983	6368	6368	6368	6368	6368
1984	11041	11041	10942	10259	10180
1985	19345	19345	18836	14382	14130
1986	33765	33765	31839	18629	18074
1987	57648	55951	50118	23763	22636
1988	94093	84036	70326	29692	27561
1989	143303	113732	88361	36346	32596
1990	199887	139408	100978	43647	37498
1991	254243	156655	106712	51328	41923
1992	297442	165447	106490	58834	45416
1993	324404	167128	101837	65493	47623
1994	333888	162230	93926	70668	48368
1995	327532	152399	84237	73885	47667
1996	308961	139630	74047	74912	45693
1997	282748	125464	64139	73780	42725
1998	253304	110877	54894	70744	39083
1999	224021	96611	46530	66212	35082
2000	196950	83193	39148	60660	30997
2001	173004	70951	32766	54555	27041
2002	152355	60056	27341	48313	23365
2003	134762	50558	22793	42257	20058
2004	119813	42420	19024	36620	17162
2005	107090	35550	15930	31541	14677
2006	96259	29818	13406	27082	12579
2007	87084	25083	11360	23246	10830
2008	79406	21200	9707	19997	9384
2009	73100	18036	8378	17280	8198
2010	68040	15471	7313	15027	7229
2011	64072	13403	6463	13173	6442
2012	61022	11742	5789	11656	5806

TABLE 7. ENGLAND AND WALES MALE POPULATION: PROJECTED TOTAL NUMBERS OF DEATHS
FROM AIDS BY END OF YEAR

basis... year	A	B	C	D	E
1983	0	0	0	0	0
1984	28	28	28	28	28
1985	124	124	124	123	123
1986	332	332	332	329	329
1987	747	747	726	732	713
1988	1537	1536	1419	1467	1361
1989	2960	2954	2563	2667	2347
1990	5436	5406	4347	4393	3657
1991	9677	9537	6982	6659	5228
1992	16755	16179	10968	9513	7170
1993	28060	26060	16873	13049	9660
1994	45021	39454	24738	17372	12718
1995	68567	55973	34273	22563	16348
1996	98601	74667	44954	28662	20517
1997	133883	94391	56188	35643	25157
1998	172401	114190	67465	43408	30160
1999	211958	133351	78391	51782	35394
2000	250636	151361	88685	60531	40714
2001	287028	167883	98164	69396	45980
2002	320281	182735	106730	78120	51069
2003	350042	195861	114348	86477	55881
2004	376335	207295	121033	94290	60346
2005	399427	217137	126836	101442	64418
2006	419694	225523	131825	107869	68080
2007	437528	232613	136085	113555	71334
2008	453291	238573	139701	118524	74196
2009	467292	243564	142759	122825	76697
2010	479798	247739	145341	126525	78869
2011	491037	251233	147520	129698	80752
2012	501210	254165	149362	132417	82381

cases of AIDS ranges from 1995 in basis C to 2000 in basis D, and the numbers of new cases in that peak year range from 21071 in 1996 in basis B to 5932 in 1998 in basis E. The peak years for deaths are a little later and the numbers are similar, whereas the peak years for new infections are much earlier, ranging from 1988 in basis C to 1993 in basis D.

It can be seen how much the results depend on the timing of the change of behaviour of homosexuals. If one could be sure that the change had taken place over 1984–1986, then the projections for the future would be generally lower than if one were to assume that significant changes did not take place until after the widespread publicity campaign during 1986–87. Evidence for the earlier date is discussed in Appendix 5 of Cox, Working Group Report (1988), but this must be taken as circumstantial, rather than conclusive.

It should be noted that the model projects numbers of cases diagnosed, rather than reported. It has been calibrated against estimates of the numbers diagnosed during the years 1984–1987. The number of cases of AIDS reported during 1988 was only 755, but it is not yet clear whether there are significant changes in reporting delays. Because of current delays in reporting, the number of cases diagnosed even for 1987 is not yet known.

TABLE 8. ENGLAND AND WALES MALE POPULATION: PROJECTED AGE-DISTRIBUTION OF NEW
CASES OF AIDS

(The numbers in the columns headed A–E are the means of the projected numbers for the end of 1986 and the end of 1987, and the age is the age at becoming sick. The numbers in the column headed compare are the actual numbers for England and Wales reported to CDSC as at 9 March 1988, and the age is the age at diagnosis. The totals may not be the sum of parts because of rounding.)

basis... age	A	B	C	D	E	compare
15–19	3	3	3	2	2	6
20–24	92	92	92	92	92	60
25–29	172	172	172	167	167	144
30–34	196	196	196	190	189	231
35–39	213	213	212	206	206	250
40–44	174	174	174	168	168	185
45–49	126	126	125	124	124	125
50–54	86	86	86	84	84	59
55–59	49	49	49	49	49	30
60–64	29	29	29	29	29	21
65+	10	10	10	10	10	32
total	1150	1150	1150	1124	1122	1143
(plus children and age unknown:						41)

Table 8 shows the projected age-distribution of new cases of AIDS somewhere in the middle of 1987, calculated as the mean of the figures at the end of 1986 and the end of 1987. These are compared with the actual age-distribution of cases of AIDS in England and Wales as reported to CDSC as at 9 March 1988. The distributions match up approximately, though far from exactly.

REFERENCES

Anderson, R. M., Medley, G. F., May, R. M. & Johnson, A. M. 1986 A preliminary study of the transmission dynamics of the Human Immunodeficiency Virus (HIV) the causative agent of AIDS. IMA J. Math. appl. Med. Biol. 3, 229–263.

Cox, D. (chairman) Department of Health Working Group 1988 Short-term prediction of HIV infection and AIDS in England and Wales. London, HMSO.

Daykin, C. D. (chairman) 1987a AIDS Working Party: AIDS Bulletin No. 1. London: Institute of Actuaries.

Daykin, C. D. (chairman) 1987b AIDS Working Party: AIDS Bulletin No. 2. London: Institute of Actuaries.

Daykin, C. D. (chairman) 1988 AIDS Working Party: AIDS Bulletin No. 3. London: Institute of Actuaries.

Daykin, C. D. (chairman) 1989 AIDS Working Party: AIDS Bulletin No. 4. London: Institute of Actuaries.

Daykin, C. D., Clark, P. N. S., Eves, M. J., Haberman, S., Le Grys, D. J., Lockyer, J., Michaelson, R. W. & Wilkie, A. D. 1988 The impact of HIV infection and AIDS on insurance in the United Kingdom. *J. Inst. Actuaries* **115**, 727–837.

Forfar, D. O., McCutcheon, J. J. & Wilkie, A. D. 1988 On graduation by mathematical formula. *J. Inst. Actuaries* **115**, 1–149.

Office of Population Censuses and Surveys 1985 Population Projections 1983–2023, series PP2, no. 13, HMSO.

Waters, H. R. & Wilkie, A. D. 1987 A short note on the construction of life tables and multiple decrement tables. *J. Inst. Actuaries* **114**, 569–580.

Wilkie, A. D. 1987 Preliminary memorandum on AIDS. Reigate, U.K.: R. Watson & Sons.

Wilkie, A. D. 1988a An actuarial model for AIDS. *Jl R. statist. Soc.* A**151**, 35–39.

Wilkie, A. D. 1988b An actuarial model for AIDS. *Occasional Actuarial Research Discussion Paper* No. 40. London: Institute of Actuaries.

Wilkie, A. D. 1988c An actuarial model for AIDS. *J. Inst. Actuaries* **115**, 839–853.

Phil. Trans. R. Soc. Lond. B **325**, 113–121 (1989)   [113]

Printed in Great Britain

ESTIMATION OF THE INCIDENCE OF HIV INFECTION

By VALERIE ISHAM

Department of Statistical Science, University College London, Gower Street,
London WC1E 6BT, U.K.

The aim of the method of 'back projection' is to provide estimates of the number of new infections with the human immunodeficiency virus (HIV) as a function of time, by using the numbers of diagnoses of the acquired immune deficiency syndrome (AIDS) together with information on the distribution of the incubation period between infection and diagnosis. Here, the method is investigated with particular reference to cases of HIV infection and AIDS in the United Kingdom.

1. INTRODUCTION

Knowledge of the prevalence of HIV infection in a particular population, and the rate at which new infections are occurring is clearly of great importance. However, for most populations of interest this information is not available. The serological data that have been collected usually relate to extremely specific groups of mostly high-risk individuals and these data cannot easily be combined to predict seroprevalence in a wider, more heterogeneous, population.

It is reasonable to suppose that new cases of HIV infection occur in a point process. For the moment we consider only those cases for which AIDS will eventually be diagnosed and denote the intensity of the corresponding point process by $h(t)$. Let the lengths of the incubation periods (between infection and diagnosis) for these individuals be independent, identically distributed variables with probability density function f. Then new diagnoses of AIDS will occur in a point process with intensity $a(t)$, where $a(t)$ is given by

$$a(t) = \int_0^\infty h(t-u) f(u) \, \mathrm{d}u. \tag{1}$$

Thus if the density of the incubation periods were known, together with the HIV infection rate $h(u)$ for $u \leqslant t$, we could calculate the distribution of the number of new diagnoses of AIDS in any time period up to time t. In many ways this would be the most natural method of predicting AIDS incidence.

Conversely, we can use equation (1) to deduce h if the functions a and f are known. This forms the basis of the method known as *back projection* in which knowledge about AIDS incidence and the distribution of incubation periods is used to make inferences about the incidence of HIV infection. It must be stressed, however, that because the proportion of those infected who will ultimately have AIDS diagnosed is not known, this method only provides information about the process of HIV infections that do subsequently lead to diagnoses of AIDS.

A related non-parametric method in discrete time of estimating the number of those already infected with HIV, which is then used to project the short-term future number of AIDS cases in the United States, is described by Brookmeyer & Gail (1986, 1988). Their work yields a lower bound on the size of the epidemic in the sense that no allowance is made for further infections.

Earlier work using back projection methods includes that of Iverson & Engen (1986) who estimate the number of those in the United States infected with HIV by blood transfusion; Rees (1987) who discusses the total numbers of those infected in the United States and in the United Kingdom, and Boldsen *et al.* (1988) who consider the total numbers of those infected in the United States and in Denmark. The assumed forms of the functions a and f can have a large influence on the estimates obtained and various possibilities have been investigated by these authors.

This paper uses the method of back projection specifically in the context of the AIDS epidemic within the population of the United Kingdom, partly to see what can be inferred about the number of individuals who have been infected with HIV over the past few years and of those who may become infected in the near future, but also to investigate the implications of specific assumptions about the functions a and f. Theoretical aspects of the method will be considered in §2 and numerical results discussed in §3.

Rates of progression from HIV infection to AIDS have been published by the Centers for Disease Control, CDC (1987). These progression rates combine the probability that an infected individual will develop AIDS with the conditional distribution of the incubation period given that AIDS is eventually diagnosed. These rates can therefore be used in a back projection calculation to produce estimates of all those infected with HIV, rather than only those ultimately developing AIDS. Results of some discrete time calculations for the United States are given in CDC (1987). The use of the CDC progression rates in the context of the epidemic in the United Kingdom is discussed in §4, whereas §5 contains some general remarks and concluding comments.

2. CONVOLUTION INVERSION IN SPECIFIC CASES

Suppose that $\tilde{a}(s)$ denotes the Fourier transform of $a(t)$,

$$\tilde{a}(s) = \int_{-\infty}^{\infty} e^{ist} a(t) \, \mathrm{d}t,$$

and similarly for $\tilde{h}(s)$ and $\tilde{f}(s)$. Then it follows immediately from (1) that

$$\tilde{a}(s) = \tilde{h}(s)\tilde{f}(s), \tag{2}$$

and therefore that $h(t)$ can be obtained by taking the inverse transform of $\tilde{a}(s)/\tilde{f}(s)$.

We shall assume some basic parametric forms for a and f. In particular, for $a(t)$ we suppose either that

$$a(t) = a_0 \exp\left(a_1 t - a_2 t^2\right), \tag{3}$$

or that

$$a(t) = (b_0 + b_1 t)\left[1 + \exp\left(b_2 - b_3 t\right)\right]^{-1} \tag{4}$$

(see Cox & Medley 1989). There are good theoretical grounds for expecting that the curve of $a(t)$ should be close to an exponential curve in the early part of the epidemic and that this rapid growth should gradually slow down as the infection spreads (see Isham (1988) for a review of mathematical models for the AIDS epidemic). Those who are at highest risk will tend to be infected early so that the epidemic will then progress more slowly amongst those who are left. The pool of those susceptible to the infection is likely gradually to diminish and behavioural changes too, will have an effect. The quadratic exponential function defined by equation (3) is a mathematically convenient way of representing a curve that, for low values of t, increases exponentially but has a slower growth rate as t increases. The linear logistic function given by equation (4) also increases exponentially for low values of t, but becomes more nearly linear for higher values of t. This curve corresponds approximately, for moderate values of t, to the solution of a fairly simple epidemic model (see Isham 1988, section 4). We do not assume that either of the functions represented by equations (3) and (4) is appropriate for arbitrarily high values of t but only over the range of values for which the form of h is to be deduced.

Two flexible parametric families of distributions have often been used to model the incubation period; the gamma distribution, denoted by $\Gamma(\alpha, \lambda)$, has density

$$f(t) = \lambda(\lambda t)^{\alpha-1} \exp(-\lambda t)/\Gamma(\alpha) \quad (t \geqslant 0), \tag{5}$$

whereas the Weibull distribution, denoted Wei (β, ρ), has density

$$f(t) = \beta\rho(\rho t)^{\beta-1} \exp[-(\rho t)^\beta] \quad (t \geqslant 0). \tag{6}$$

See, for example, Lui et al. (1986); Blythe & Anderson (1988); Medley et al. (1987); Anderson & Medley (1988); Giesecke et al. (1988) and Lui et al. (1988) for discussion on modelling the incubation period distribution.

If $a(t)$ is given by equation (3) then

$$\tilde{a}(s) = a_0(\pi/a_2)^{\frac{1}{2}} \exp[(a_1+is)^2/(4a_2)]. \tag{7}$$

The gamma distribution (equation (5)) also has a simple Fourier transform and it is straightforward to check that in this case $h(t)$ satisfies

$$h(t) = a_0 \exp[a_1^2/(4a_2)][1-(2a_2/\lambda)D_{a_1}]^\alpha \exp[-(a_1-2a_2 t)^2/(4a_2)], \tag{8}$$

where D_{a_1} is the partial differential operator, with respect to a_1. In particular we have

$$h(t)/a(t) = \begin{cases} x(t) & \alpha = 1 \\ x^2(t)-2a_2/\lambda^2 & \alpha = 2 \\ x^3(t)-6a_2 x(t)/\lambda^2 & \alpha = 3 \\ x^4(t)-12a_2 x^2(t)/\lambda^2+12a_2^2/\lambda^4 & \alpha = 4 \end{cases} \tag{9}$$

where $x(t) = 1+(a_1-2a_2 t)/\lambda$, $x^n(t) \equiv [x(t)]^n$ and $a(t)$ is given in equation (3).

If we choose to use the Weibull distribution (6) for the incubation periods, then analytic determination of $h(t)$ by using equation (2) is not feasible and we proceed numerically. A simple method that can be used if the index β of the Weibull distribution is a (small) integer is the following, which we describe for the case $\beta = 2$. First, write equation (1) in the alternative form

$$a(t) = \int_{-\infty}^t h(u)f(t-u)\,\mathrm{d}u. \tag{10}$$

On differentiating twice with respect to t, we obtain the integral equation

$$a''(t) = h(t)f'(0) + \int_{-\infty}^t h(u)f''(t-u)\,\mathrm{d}u, \tag{11}$$

where $a'(t) = \mathrm{d}a(t)/\mathrm{d}t$, $a''(t) = \mathrm{d}^2a(t)/\mathrm{d}t^2$ and so on. Since for $\beta = 2$, $f'(0) = 2\rho^2 \neq 0$, equation (11) is a Volterra equation of the second kind that can be solved by a process of successive approximation, yielding a numerical evaluation of $h(t)$ for known functions a and f (Tricomi 1957, chapter 1). This method is widely applicable and is not restricted to the particular functions given by equations (3) or (4), together with equation (6) with which we are concerned here.

3. NUMERICAL RESULTS

The functions $f(t)$ and $a(t)$ are the rates at which infections with HIV and diagnoses of AIDS occur. Thus the expected numbers of infections and diagnoses in any particular time period can be obtained by integrating these rates appropriately. We shall take time measured in units of one year, with $t = 0$ corresponding to the start of 1979, and denote by $H_i(A_i)$ the expected incidences of infections (diagnoses) in year i. Thus

$$H_i = \int_{i-1979}^{i-1978} h(u)\,\mathrm{d}u, \tag{12}$$

and similarly for A_i.

The functions $a(t)$ given by equations (3) and (4) have been fitted by Cox & Medley (1989) to AIDS diagnosis data for the United Kingdom reported up to June 1988. The parameter estimates obtained are as follows:

equation (3) quadratic exponential:

$$a_0 = 0.08073 \quad a_1 = 1.6447 \quad a_2 = 0.06558,$$

equation (4) linear logistic:

$$b_0 = 77.645 \quad b_1 = 176.117 \quad b_2 = 6.871 \quad b_3 = 0.8233.$$

It must be emphasized that the standard errors attached to these parameter estimates are relatively large and that the fitted values A_i are sensitive to small changes in the estimates, especially in a_2 (Cox & Medley 1989).

For the years 1980–1993, the expected numbers of diagnoses, A_i, corresponding to these curves are tabulated in table 1. Over the period 1980–1987 the values of A_i for the linear logistic curve are very close to those for the quadratic exponential curve. After 1987, the approach to linearity of the former values starts to appear in contrast to the latter values that peak and then begin to decrease.

TABLE 1. EXPECTED ANNUAL INCIDENCE OF AIDS DIAGNOSES, A_i

year i	quadratic exponential	linear logistic
1980	1	1
1981	4	5
1982	12	13
1983	36	37
1984	97	94
1985	227	225
1986	465	470
1987	838	840
1988	1327	1261
1989	1845	1644
1990	2252	1954
1991	2416	2206
1992	2276	2420
1993	1883	2614

In each case the rate of diagnoses $a(t)$ is given by equations (3) or (4); the parameter values are as given earlier; A_i is obtained by integrating $a(t)$ over the appropriate year.

Anderson & Medley (1988) fitted both the gamma and Weibull distributions, given by equations (5) and (6) respectively, for the incubation period using data for transfusion recipients available up to April 1988, together with a parametric model for the rate at which infected transfusions took place, and obtained the parameter estimates; $\Gamma(\alpha, \lambda)$, $\alpha = 2.70$, $\lambda = 0.19$, (mean 14.3); Wei (β, ρ), $\beta = 2.33$, $\rho = 0.12$, (mean 7.4).

For numerical convenience we shall compare expected annual incidence of HIV infections, H_i, assuming the incubation periods have either the $\Gamma(2, 0.14)$, $\Gamma(3, 0.21)$ or Wei $(2, 0.12)$ distributions that have means 14.3, 14.3 or 7.4 respectively. The Weibull and gamma distributions with index 2 will be used to calculate values of H_i with both forms for $a(t)$. Results using the gamma distribution with index 3 will only be given when $a(t)$ has the quadratic exponential form. Values of H_i for all these cases are given in table 2.

TABLE 2. EXPECTED ANNUAL INCIDENCE OF HIV INFECTIONS, H_i

| $f(t)...$ | $\Gamma(3, 0.21)$ | $\Gamma(2, 0.14)$ | | Wei $(2, 0.12)$ | |
$a(t)...$	quadratic exponential	quadratic exponential	linear logistic	quadratic exponential	linear logistic
year, i					
1980	365	106	123	62	71
1981	1083	348	347	201	196
1982	2741	980	912	556	514
1983	5830	2364	2242	1320	1255
1984	10273	4851	4935	2652	2725
1985	14544	8366	8918	4455	4784
1986	15488	11877	11592	6110	5845
1987	9945	13312	9492	6516	4188
1988	−2076	10546	4940	4726	1822
1989	−15499	3198	2685	895	1462
1990	−22669	−6226	2830	−3320	2470
1991	−19244	−13394	3649	−5674	3464
1992	−8016	−15036	4351	−4997	4029
1993	3489	−11208	4836	−2101	4265
total 1980–1987 inclusive	60269	42204	38561	21872	19578

There are a number of points to note. Firstly, negative values of H_i are obtained in later years when the quadratic exponential function is used for $a(t)$, which means that this function is not compatible with the various assumed incubation period distributions over the whole 1980–1993 time period. Essentially, in such cases, if the early values of $h(t)$ are determined to give the quadratic exponential function $a(t)$ for low values of t, then too many AIDS diagnoses will occur later. To compensate for these, negative numbers of infections are then needed if the function $a(t)$ is to have the chosen increasing doubling time. When $a(t)$ has the linear logistic form, no negative values of H_i are obtained over the 1980–1993 time period, although there is still an implausible oscillation in the later values. However, the function $a(t)$ has been fitted using data only up to June 1988 and only the lower tail of the incubation period distribution curve can be fitted. This lack of compatibility is not therefore surprising. On the other hand, the figures for expected HIV incidence up to 1986 might be hoped to be reasonably reliable. Note also that the similarity between the fitted values for the two forms of $a(t)$ up to 1987 results in a corresponding similarity in the values of H_i up to 1986 (using a particular distribution for the incubation periods).

Secondly, with the assumption of the gamma distribution, $\Gamma(2, 0.14)$ or $\Gamma(3, 0.21)$, only 41% or 35% respectively of incubation periods will be of length 10 years or less, as compared with 76% for the Weibull distribution. Thus the annual incidence of HIV infection with either of the gamma distributions must be much higher than that using the Weibull distribution during the early stages of an epidemic, to produce the same function $a(t)$. If we compare the total numbers of HIV infections occurring during 1980–1987 given in table 2, we see that the totals for the gamma distributions are almost double, or more, those for the Weibull distribution.

Thirdly, it is of interest to note that the use of an exponential curve for $a(t)$ with no quadratic term, together with the Weibull distribution for the incubation period, results in a total of some 22000 HIV infections over the years 1980–1987. This number is very similar to those obtained using the quadratic exponential or linear logistic curves although the numbers in individual years follow a different pattern.

4. THE CDC PROGRESSION RATES

In a paper by the Centers for Disease Control (1987), estimates of progression rates to AIDS are given based on data for a subgroup of HIV-positive men taking part in the San Francisco City Clinic Cohort Study. (There is apparently an error in the rates quoted that has been corrected in rates given by Curran *et al.* (1988).) Thus if p_i is the probability that an infected individual develops AIDS between i and $i+1$ years after infection, estimates of p_i, $i = 0, \ldots, 9$ are as given in table 3.

TABLE 3. PROBABILITIES OF PROGRESSION FROM HIV INFECTION TO AIDS

(p_i, CDC estimate of the probability of developing AIDS between i and $i+1$ years after infection; F_i, probability of incubation period of length between i and $i+1$ years, for Wei (2, 0.12).)

years after infection, i	0	1	2	3	4	5	6	7	8	9	total $i = 0, \ldots, 9$
$100 p_i$	0	2	3	5	5	9	6	6	6	5	47
$100 F_i$	1	4	7	8	10	10	10	10	9	7	76
$100 \times (47/76) F_i$	1	2	4	5	6	6	6	6	6	4	

It follows that an estimated 47% of all those infected will have had AIDS diagnosed within 10 years of infection. Note that these probabilities are not conditional upon the event that an infected individual does eventually have AIDS diagnosed. If this latter event has probability p, and if F_i is the probability that an incubation period has a length between i and $i+1$ years, then $p_i = pF_i$. For comparison, the values of F_i for the Wei (2, 0.12) distribution are also given in table 3, rounded to the nearest hundredth.

If p were to be $47/76 \approx 0.6$, then the values of pF_i for this Weibull distribution, again given to the nearest 1% in table 3, are broadly similar to the CDC values p_i.

A discrete time approximation to equation (1) by using a year as the unit of time is

$$A_i = \sum_{j=0}^{\infty} H_{i-j} F_j = (1/p) \sum_{j=0}^{\infty} H_{i-j} p_j. \tag{13}$$

For a given set of values $\{A_i\}$ with the year i going back to the start of the epidemic, and a set of p_i values as in table 3, equation (13) can be used to deduce the corresponding values of H_i/p; these are estimates of the annual incidence of all infections with HIV regardless of whether or not these lead to subsequent diagnoses of AIDS. For example, using the annual AIDS incidence A_i for the quadratic exponential model given in table 1 (the corresponding A_{1979} is 0) with the CDC values p_i from table 3, we obtain the values of H_i/p listed in table 4.

TABLE 4. EXPECTED ANNUAL INCIDENCE OF ALL HIV INFECTIONS, H_i/p, USING THE
QUADRATIC EXPONENTIAL MODEL AND THE CDC PROGRESSION PROBABILITIES

year, i	1979	1980	1981	1982	1983	1984	1985	1986	1987
H_i/p	50	125	288	931	2197	4295	7168	9339	9640
$(47/76)H_i/p$	31	77	178	576	1359	2656	4433	5775	5962

Note that values of H_i/p for i after 1987 cannot be deduced until estimates of p_i for $i > 9$ are available. Also, as is to be expected given the similarities noted in table 4, scaling the H_i/p values by the factor $47/76$ gives a set of values that closely resemble the H_i values obtained in table 2 using the Weibull distribution, again with the quadratic exponential function $a(t)$. Use of the linear logistic curve in place of the quadratic exponential curve in the above calculations gives very similar results over this time period, since the values of A_i up to 1987 are almost identical for the two curves.

5. DISCUSSION

The analytic forms for the rate, $a(t)$, of AIDS diagnoses and the density, $f(t)$, of the incubation period have been chosen and their parameters fitted using data currently available and therefore necessarily lying within restricted ranges of values of t. In particular, information is only available about the shape of the lower part of the distribution curve for the incubation period. Inevitably, then, the predicted values of the rate, $h(t)$, of HIV infection (or the annual incidence, H_i, of HIV infection) obtained by using values of $a(t)$ or $f(t)$ for t lying outside these ranges must be treated with great caution. Even up to 1987 the projected values of H_i vary considerably with the particular incubation period distribution used.

I have already noted the broad similarity in shape between the estimated probabilities p_i given by CDC (1987) and the corresponding discretized Weibull distribution $\{F_i\}$ given in table 3. If one were to believe that these sets of probabilities are approximately correct then one would be led to an estimate of around 0.6 for the probability p that an HIV infected individual will subsequently be diagnosed as having AIDS. It appears from table 2 that, assuming the Weibull distribution for incubation periods, the total number of HIV infections in the United Kingdom between 1980 and 1987 inclusive, which will lead to subsequent diagnoses of AIDS, is perhaps of the order of 20–22 000. If we include all HIV infections, not just those leading to AIDS diagnoses, the corresponding range could be 33–37 000 (if the entries in table 2 are scaled by a factor of 10/6). To be more specific it will be necessary to examine further the relative merits of the parametric forms for $a(t)$ and $f(t)$ that have been used.

It is self-evident that projections of this sort are entirely dependent on the assumptions being made. If the functions a and f were known then the HIV infection rate h could be determined exactly from equation (1). Error in the assumed forms of a or f will be reflected in errors in the estimated annual incidence of HIV infection, H_i. In some cases the assumed forms will be clearly incompatible, at least over part of their ranges, as is apparent from the negative values of H_i given in table 2 which obtain when $a(t)$ has the quadratic exponential form. The linear logistic curve for $a(t)$ gives more satisfactory results although, as remarked earlier, the oscillation in H_i does not seem entirely plausible.

One source of error that has been suggested is that whereas the population being considered is the whole population of the United Kingdom with $a(t)$ being fitted to all AIDS diagnoses in those countries, the incubation period distributions fitted by Anderson & Medley (1988) were obtained by using data on recipients of blood transfusions. The CDC probabilities refer to those (presumably) infected by homosexual transmission. It might be expected that the distribution of the length of the incubation period would vary with the mode of transmission. That $a(t)$ is the total rate of AIDS diagnoses summed over all risk groups is not a problem in the method described in this paper for inferring the rate of HIV infection, as long as the density f of incubation periods is an appropriately weighted mixture of distributions applying to each risk group separately. In particular, the fitted Weibull distribution could be inappropriate for the majority of AIDS cases that have occurred so far. The weights used in combining the distributions might need to change with time as the infection starts to spread into different subgroups of the population (grouped for example by risk or by spatial considerations). Were the necessary data available, back projection of HIV incidence for each subgroup separately would avoid this problem. However, recent work by Anderson & Medley (1988) and Lui *et al.* (1988) suggests that the mode of transmission of infection does not have a strong effect on the distribution of the incubation period and so the assumption of a common incubation period distribution is not too unreasonable as a first approximation. There is also evidence (Darby *et al.* 1989) that the incubation period distribution does vary with the age of the infected individual, but again this is not a problem as long as f is the appropriately weighted mixture of such distributions.

I am grateful to Roy Anderson, F.R.S., David Cox, F.R.S., and Graham Medley for providing me with prepublication copies of their papers and for helpful discussion.

REFERENCES

Anderson, R. M. & Medley, G. F. 1988 Epidemiology, HIV infection and AIDS: the incubation and infectious periods, survival and vertical transmission. *AIDS* **2**, S57–S63.

Blythe, S. P. & Anderson, R. M. 1988 Distributed incubation and infectious periods in models of the transmission dynamics of the human immunodeficiency virus (HIV). *IMA J. Math. appl. med. Biol.* **5**, 1–19.

Boldsen, J. L., Jensen, J. L., Søgaard, J. & Sorensen, M. 1988 On the incubation time distribution and the Danish AIDS data. *J. R. statist. Soc.* A **151**, 42–43.

Brookmeyer, R. & Gail, M. H. 1986 The minimum size of the AIDS epidemic in the United States. Lancet(ii), 1320–1322.

Brookmeyer, R. & Gail, M. H. 1988 A method for obtaining short term projections and lower bounds on the size of the AIDS epidemic. *J. Am. statist. Ass.* **83**, 301–308.

Centers for Disease Control 1987 Human immunodeficiency virus infection in the United States: a review of current knowledge. *MMWR* **36** (suppl. no. S-6), 1–48.

Cox, D. R. & Medley, G. F. 1989 A process of events with notification delay and the forecasting of AIDS. *Phil. Trans. R. Soc. Lond.* B **325**, 135–145. (This issue.)

Curran, J. W., Jaffe, H. W., Hardy, A. M., Meade Morgan, W., Selik, R. M. & Dondero, T. J. 1988 Epidemiology of HIV infection and AIDS in the United States. *Science, Wash.* **239**, 610–616.

Darby, S. C., Rizza, C. R., Doll, R., Spooner, R. J., Stratton, I. M. & Thakrar, B. 1989 Incidence of AIDS and excess mortality associated with HIV in haemophiliacs in the U.K. *Br. med. J.* **298**, 1064–1068.

Giesecke, J., Scalia-Tomba, G., Berglund, O., Berntorp, E., Schulman, S. & Stigendal, L. 1988 Incidence of symptoms and AIDS in 146 Swedish haemophiliacs and blood transfusion recipients infected with human immunodeficiency virus. *Br. med. J.* **297**, 99–102.

Isham, V. 1988 Mathematical modelling of the transmission dynamics of HIV infection and AIDS: a review. *J. R. statist. Soc.* A **151**, 5–49.

Iversen, O.-J. & Engen, S. 1986 Epidemiology of AIDS — statistical analyses. *J. Epidemiol. Commnty Hlth*, **41**, 55–58.

Lui, K-J., Lawrence, D. N.,, Morgan, W. M., Peterman, T. A., Haverkos, H. W. & Bregman, D. J. 1986 A model-based approach for estimating the mean incubation period of transfusion-associated acquired immunodeficiency syndrome. *Proc. natn. Acad. Sci. U.S.A.*, **83**, 3051–3055.

Lui, K-J., Darrow, W. W. & Rutherford, G. W. III 1988 A model based estimate of the mean incubation period for AIDS in homosexual men. *Science, Wash.* **240**, 1333–1335.

Medley, G. F., Anderson, R. M., Cox, D. R. & Billard, L. 1987 Incubation period of AIDS in patients infected via blood transfusion. *Nature, Lond.* **328**, 718–721.

Rees, M. 1987 The sombre view of AIDS. *Nature, Lond.* **326**, 343–345.

Tricomi, F. G. 1957 *Integral equations.* New York: Wiley Interscience.

Note added in proof – 22 May 1989

The recent issue of *Statistics in Medicine* (1989, **8**, part 1) devoted entirely to AIDS modelling, contains several papers describing the use of the back-projection method in connection with the AIDS epidemic in the U.S.A. In particular, Brookmeyer & Damiano (1989) extend earlier work by Brookmeyer & Gail (1988), and Taylor (1989) uses a similar approach. De Gruttola & Lagakos discuss problems arising from uncertainty about the appropriate form for $h(t)$.

References

Brookmeyer, R. & Damiano, A. 1989 Statistical methods for short-term predictions of the AIDS incidence. *Statist. Med.* **8**, 23–34.

De Gruttola, V. & Lagakos, S. W. 1989 The value of AIDS incidence data in assessing the spread of HIV infection. *Statist. Med.* **8**, 35–44.

Taylor, J. H. G. 1989 Models for the HIV infection and AIDS epidemic in the United States. *Statist. Med.* **8**, 45–58.

Phil. Trans. R. Soc. Lond. B **325**, 123–134 (1989)   [123]

Printed in Great Britain

PREDICTIONS OF THE AIDS EPIDEMIC IN THE U.K.: THE USE OF THE BACK PROJECTION METHOD

By N. E. DAY, S. M. GORE, M. A. McGEE and M. SOUTH

MRC Biostatistics Unit, 5 Shaftesbury Road, Cambridge CB2 2BW, U.K.

Back projection methods are used to predict the yearly number of new AIDS diagnoses and the number of new HIV infections, to the end of 1992. The AIDS, but not the HIV, predictions are insensitive to the choice of incubation period distribution. A wide range of predictions is consistent with the AIDS diagnoses in years up to 1987, but limited ancillary information on the relative rates of new HIV infection in 1984 to 1987 can be used to narrow this range. The range of prediction based on AIDS reports to the end of 1988 is lower and narrower than the range based on reports to the end of 1987. The number of new AIDS cases in 1992 appears likely to fall in the range 1000–3000.

1. INTRODUCTION

Accuracy in predicting the future of the AIDS epidemic depends on the extent of the information on which the predictions are based. Methods range from those that simply use the number of reported AIDS cases, to those that model the full dynamics of transmission in the population. The former are arithmetic exercises in extrapolation ignoring whatever is known of the epidemiology of the disease, and cannot incorporate information that one might have on changing patterns of transmission. They are reliable in the very short term, but are also likely to be overtaken by events; even in the medium term, the predictions may prove wildly inaccurate. Methods that model the full dynamics of the epidemic can provide much insight into the qualitative evolution of the epidemic, and identify the key variables that determine in the short and medium terms the number of cases that occur. Accurate information on these variables is, however, sparse and very difficult to obtain. Intermediate between these two approaches to prediction is the back projection method (Brookmeyer & Davison 1988; Zeger *et al.* 1989). The advantage of this method for short and medium term projections is that it can utilize the available information of particular importance for predicting the number of AIDS cases, namely the number of new HIV infections up to the present. Precise information on HIV infection is lacking, and a major epidemiological challenge is to construct ways of acquiring it in the future. Some data are available and these can be used to assess the credibility of different possible projections.

Back projection is based on the underlying relation between the number of new cases of AIDS in time t to $t + dt$, which we designate $a(t)$, and the number of new HIV infections $h(s)$ at each time s since the start of the epidemic ($s = 0$) through the incubation period distribution $f(u)$, u being the time spent between initial infection and diagnosis of AIDS:

$$a(t) = \int_0^t h(s) f(t-s) \, ds. \tag{1}$$

If one knew $f(u)$, then this relation could be inverted to express $h(s)$ for all $0 \leqslant s \leqslant t$

as a function of $a(s)$, $0 \leqslant s \leqslant t$. More generally we can construct a family of values for $h(s)$, $0 \leqslant s \leqslant t$, which are consistent with a particular realization of $a(s)$, $0 \leqslant s \leqslant t$.

For practical purposes, the time axis will be grouped into intervals $(t_0(=0), t_1)$, (t_1, t_2) to (t_{n-1}, t_n). We designate by a_i and h_i the number of new AIDS cases and HIV infections respectively in the time interval (t_{i-1}, t_i), $i = 1, \ldots, n$.

We then have an approximate discrete version of relation (1),

$$a_i = \sum_{j=1}^{i} h_j f_{i-j}, \tag{2}$$

where

$$f_{i-j} = \int_{t_{i-j}}^{t_{i-j+1}} f(u) \, du,$$

or

$$\boldsymbol{a}_i = F_i \boldsymbol{h}_i,$$

where

$$\boldsymbol{a}_i = (a_1, \ldots, a_i), \boldsymbol{h}_i = (h_1, \ldots, h_i)$$

and F_i is the appropriate matrix.

The k, jth element of F_i will be given by

$$f_{kj} = f_{k-j} \quad (k \geqslant j)$$

$$= 0 \quad (k < j).$$

We then have

$$\boldsymbol{h}_i = F_i^{-1} \boldsymbol{a}_i$$

where F_i^{-1} has the same form as F_i, i.e.

$$f_{kj}^{(-1)} = f_{k-j}^{(-1)} \quad (k \geqslant j)$$

$$= 0 \quad (k < j)$$

with the $f_{k-j}^{(-1)}$ given straight forwardly by

$$f_0 f_k^{(-1)} = -\sum_{m=1}^{k} f_m f_{k-m}^{(-1)} \quad (k > 0)$$

and

$$f_0 f_0^{(-1)} = 1.$$

2. MATERIALS AND METHODS

We assume a certain form for the incubation period distribution $f(t)$. Then on the basis of observed values of $a(t)$ up to the present, we calculate the range of values of $h(t)$ consistent with the observed $a(t)$. This range of values of $h(t)$ is then examined in the light of available knowledge on HIV infection in the population, limited and mostly indirect, but nevertheless sufficient to indicate that some of the range of values for $h(t)$ are implausible.

Predictions of future AIDS cases are made by projecting forwards from the HIV estimates, by using the incubation period distribution. Assumptions have to be made regarding future HIV infections. The importance of these assumptions for future AIDS cases is examined, and their plausibility assessed in terms of the weak available data on trends in HIV infection.

Available data

(i) *Number of AIDS cases*

Our analysis is based on AIDS cases among U.K. residents. The biologically meaningful measure for the number of AIDS cases is the number of new diagnoses, in suitably chosen time intervals. The monthly published figures refer to reports, not diagnoses, and the delay between the two is variable. The Communicable Disease Surveillance Centre (CDSC) has made available a tape giving information on all reports to 30 June 1988 that includes date of diagnosis (table 1 a). The number of reports, with no further information, is available for each month to the end of 1988 (table 1 c). By using data on reports up to the end of 1987, and assuming an exponential increase in the epidemic for 1988 and 1989, the figures in column 1 of table 2 for the number of AIDS diagnoses in each year from 1982 to 1987 are produced (Healy 1988). We refer to these as the earlier Healy estimates for 1987. Data on reports to the end of 1988 make these estimates untenable (table 1 a and 1 c).

TABLE 1. YEARLY REPORTS AND DIAGNOSES OF AIDS

(a) Year of diagnosis and year of report for AIDS cases reported[a] to mid 1988.

year of diagnosis

year of report	total	1982	1983	1984	1985	1986	1987	1988	unknown
1982	2	2	—	—	—	—	—	—	0
1983	26[b]	4	19	—	—	—	—	—	0
1984	76[c]	3	9	61	—	—	—	—	2
1985	156	1	1	29	117	—	—	—	8
1986	298	1	0	10	63	216	—	—	8
1987	612	0	3	1	40	165	402	—	1
Jan.–Jun. 1988	362	0	0	1	2	23	129	202	5
total	1532	11	32	102	222	404	531	202	24
Imputed year of diagnosis for the 24 unknowns	—	—	6	10	4	3	1	—

(b) Distribution of reporting delays for the 362 cases reported in the first half of 1988.

report delay (months)	0	1–3	4–6	7–9	10–12	13–18	19–24	25–29
probability	0.194	0.497	0.126	0.070	0.020	0.045	0.037	0.011

(c) Empirical assignation of year of diagnosis, for cases reported from July 1988.

Empirically assigned year of diagnosis

year of report	total	1986	1987	1988
Jly–Dec. 1988	393	11.6	39.4	341.9
Jan.–Jun. 1989[d]	419	2.5	26.8	146.5
Jly–Dec. 1989[d]	445	—	13.0	44.5
Jan.–Jun. 1990[d]	471	—	2.8	30.1
Jly–Dec. 1990[d]	497	—	—	14.6
total	2225	14.1	82.0	577.6

[a] Excludes visitors to U.K.
[b] Includes three diagnosed in 1981.
[c] Includes one diagnosed in 1979.
[d] Imputation based on linear extrapolation of quarterly report totals for 1987 and 1988, namely 137, 138, 182, 155, 199, 163, 199 and 194.

We take a different approach. For the 18 months to the end of 1988, the number of new AIDS reports per quarter has remained nearly constant. The number of new reports in each quarter of 1989 and 1990 has been estimated by linear extrapolation from the results for July 1987 to December 1988. The observed delay distribution for cases reported in the first 6 months of 1988 is given in table 1 b. The distribution is truncated at 30 months.

Applying the backward delay distribution of table 1 b to these extrapolated figures yields the year of diagnosis as given in table 1 c. We have also allocated proportionally a year of diagnosis for the 24 cases in table 1 a for which year of report diagnosis was unknown. The final figures for the yearly number of AIDS diagnoses that we have used in the remainder of the paper are given in the second column of table 2; they incorporate the further data from CDSC to the end of 1988. Up to 1986 the first two columns of table 2 are, of course, nearly identical. The second column figure for 1987 depends little on our assumption for reports in 1989 and seems likely to be near the truth. The figure for 1988 is more speculative. Our principal predictions for AIDS cases per year up to 1992 are based on our current estimates of yearly AIDS diagnoses from 1982 to 1987 inclusive.

TABLE 2. ESTIMATED NUMBER OF AIDS DIAGNOSES BY YEAR

year	earlier estimate, based on reports to Dec. 1987	current estimate, based on reports to Dec. 1988
1982	10	11
1983	30	32
1984	109	108
1985	224	232
1986	425	426
1987	762	610
1988	—	777

(ii) *Incubation period distribution*

Three different distributions have been used, two based on fitting Weibull and Gamma distributions to observed data and the third, which we call the CDC distribution, based on observed empirical distribution (table 3). In the period of interest, the CDC distribution is close to twice the gamma; half the CDC distribution is shown in table 3 and has been used in further computation. In fact predictions up to 1992, based on reports to the end of 1988, are not sensitive to changes in the incubation period distribution. (The extent to which predictions further into the future are affected by this distribution is the subject of a separate paper.) Without this lack of sensitivity in short-term AIDS forecasts the method would be questionable since the progression of HIV disease is known to be heterogeneous across different subgroups of the population.

(iii) *Assumptions about the number of HIV infecteds in the population, by year*

Our aim is to explore a range of probabilistic evolutions of the number of cases of HIV infection over time that are consistent with, (i) the number of AIDS cases reported to the end of 1988, from which is derived the number of AIDS diagnoses to the end of 1987, and (ii) available data on HIV prevalence in previous years, albeit incomplete and from selected subsamples.

TABLE 3. PROGRESSION RATES FOR DIFFERENT INCUBATION PERIOD DISTRIBUTIONS

new percentage (cumulative %) progressing to AIDS after t years

incubation distribution, $t =$	1	2	3	4	5	6	7	8	9	10	11	12	total at 10 years
Gamma	0.3	0.9 (1.2)	1.6 (2.8)	2.2 (5.0)	2.7 (7.7)	3.0 (10.7)	3.3 (14.0)	3.5 (17.5)	3.6 (21.1)	3.7 (24.8)	3.7 (28.5)	3.7 (32.2)	24.8
$\frac{1}{2} \times$ CDC rates (extrapolated from Gamma)	0	1.0 (1.0)	1.5 (2.5)	2.5 (5.0)	2.5 (7.5)	4.5 (12.0)	3.0 (15.0)	3.0 (18.0)	3.0 (21.0)	2.5 (23.5)	5.0 (28.5)	3.7 (32.2)	23.5
CDC rates (extrapolated from 2 × Gamma)	0	2.0 (2.0)	3.0 (5.0)	5.0 (10.0)	5.0 (15.0)	9.0 (24.0)	6.0 (30.0)	6.0 (36.0)	6.0 (42.0)	5.0 (47.0)	10.0 (57.0)	7.4 (64.4)	47.0
Weibull	0.3	2.8 (3.1)	5.4 (8.5)	7.5 (16.0)	9.0 (25.0)	9.9 (34.9)	10.2 (45.1)	9.9 (55.0)	9.1 (64.1)	8.1 (72.2)	6.8 (79.0)	5.6 (84.6)	72.2

[89]

We have assumed that $h(t)$, the number of new infections in time t to $t+dt$, can be described as
$$h(t) = a\exp{(bt+ct^2)}, \text{with } t = 0 \text{ at January } 1981.$$

In expression (2), we have taken as an approximation to h_i the weighted sum: $\frac{1}{4}h(i-1)+\frac{1}{2}h(i-\frac{1}{2})+\frac{1}{4}h(i)$. This functional form produces some improbable extrapolations to years beyond 1990; we have used it as a means of exploring different forms of the epidemic of HIV infection up to the present. In particular, we examined continuing exponential increase in the number of new cases of HIV infection per year in comparison to a slowing of the rate of increase, and a maximum reached somewhere between 1984 and 1988. There is considerable evidence that the risk behaviour of homosexual men has changed; changes, which may have begun in 1983, were widespread in 1985 and continued in 1986 and 1987 (Johnson & Gill 1988). This suggests that large increases in the yearly number of HIV-positives did not occur from 1985 to 1988, and that there may well have been a fall.

(iv) *Model fitting*

For each assumed incubation period distribution, by computation over a three dimensional grid, the range of values of a, b and c was determined for which the predicted number of AIDS cases in years 1982 to 1987 were consistent with the observed, using as a consistency measure a goodness of fit X^2 on 6 degrees of freedom (90% point). Additional fits were made including the preliminary estimates of 1988 AIDS diagnoses, and also to the numbers (column 1 of table 2) assumed in earlier reports (referred to as the earlier estimates).

For each set of values for a, b and c, the expected number of AIDS cases, and new HIV infections, were calculated for each year to 1992. The set of values of a, b and c consistent with the 1982–87 AIDS data generates a range of values for predicted numbers, both of new cases in 1992 and the cumulative number of cases up to the end of 1992.

Many of the values for a, b and c that generate expected AIDS cases consistent with the data to the end of 1987 generate implausible numbers of new HIV infecteds in the years 1985 to 1988, implausible either because they show a rapid rise or too rapid a decline. The crucial value in this respect is given by the time to peak HIV incidence, t_p, where $t_p = -b/2c$. If t_p is less than 3, there are unrealistically few new infections in 1987 and 1988; if t_p is greater than 8, then 1988 new infections are largely in excess of those of 1985.

3. RESULTS

The incubation period distributions shown in table 3 range from less than 25% progression in 10 years for the gamma and half-CDC to nearly 75% for the Weibull. The CDC distribution is intermediate, and predictions were initially based on it. By using the current estimates of yearly AIDS diagnoses to the end of 1987, the range of predicted AIDS cases in 1992 is from 737 to 3538. The parameter values that best fit the data to 1987 predict 1031 AIDS cases in 1992. Table 4 gives the predictions by year, for both new AIDS cases and new HIV infections. Both the extreme low and the extreme high seem unlikely. For the former, it is very improbable that so few new infections would have occurred in 1987 and 1988, and none in later years. It is interesting, however, that such results are consistent with the current data on AIDS cases. The 'extreme high' model proposes a doubling of the number of new HIV infecteds between 1985 and 1988; this conflicts with what is known of changing behaviour.

TABLE 4. PREDICTED NEW AIDS CASES AND NEW HIV INFECTEDS BY YEAR TO 1992

(AIDS cases, current estimates for 1987; assumed incubation distribution, CDC rates.)

	1987 current estimate	AIDS cases predictions to 1992			HIV infecteds predictions to 1992		
		best fit	lowest	highest	best fit	lowest	highest
1981	—	—	—	—	410	307	724
1982	11	8	6	14	1233	1349	1212
1983	32	37	36	46	2575	3097	1935
1984	108	109	118	111	3732	3727	2945
1985	232	234	250	214	3756	2353	4274
1986	426	414	409	396	2625	778	5914
1987	610	616	567	643	1273	134	7802
1988	—	809	708	985	428	12	9813
1989	—	955	781	1437	100	1	11767
1990	—	1021	763	2002	16	0	13453
1991	—	1031	726	2717	2	0	14664
1992	—	1031	737	3538	0	0	15239
predicted total to 1992		6265	5101	12103	16150	11758	89742
t_p = time to peak HIV incidence; $t = 0$ = Jan. 1981					4.02	3.29	11.81

Table 5 compares predictions based on the CDC incubation period distribution to those based on the Weibull (faster progression) and on the half-CDC (slower progression). There is a major difference in the predicted numbers of HIV infecteds, the approximately 3-fold difference between prediction based on the Weibull and the half-CDC reflecting the similar proportional difference between the two distributions, up to 12 years. Both the best estimate and the range of predictions for the yearly number of AIDS cases to 1992 are similar for the three distributions.

The range of predictions for the number of new AIDS cases in 1992 is related to the different forms of the HIV epidemic model from which the AIDS cases are derived, specifically in terms of the time t_p at which the HIV epidemic is assumed to have peaked. This relation is shown in table 6a; table 7 illustrates the form that the HIV epidemic is assumed to take for a range of values of t_p. This table demonstrates three points: first, that knowing the number of new infections, by year, greatly improves the precision of the predictions of new HIV cases; second, that crude and unsystematic information, as described by Johnson & Gill (1988), can be used at least to assign plausibilities to the different values in table 6; and third, that reliable information on new HIV infections would be valuable for estimating the incubation period distribution, even if all data were anonymous.

The values in table 7 are for the CDC distribution. Values generated by the Weibull and the half-CDC distribution are proportionately almost exactly the same, but smaller or larger by a factor of 1.5 approximately in absolute value respectively. The form assumed for the course of the HIV epidemic has three parameters, of which t_p only fixes one. For given t_p, the range of values for the other two parameters, which are consistent with the observed AIDS data, is small.

Figure 1 displays graphically the information of tables 4–7. One can see the insensitivity of the 1992 AIDS prediction to the assumed form of the incubation period distribution, and the sensitivity of the HIV-infected estimates. The relation between the time point at which HIV infection is assumed to have peaked and the 1992 AIDS predictions is also clear.

In table 5, we also study the effect of accumulating additional information on AIDS diagnoses on short and medium term AIDS predictions. We consider the situation as it was in early 1988,

TABLE 5. CUMULATIVE HIV INFECTEDS BY THE END OF 1987 AND PREDICTED NEW AIDS CASES IN 1988 AND 1992

| incubation distribution | observed AIDS data | best fit predictions | | | | extremes consistent with data | | | | | | | |
| | | | | | | low | | | | high | | | |
		1981–1987 HIV	1988 AIDS	1992 AIDS	t_p	1981–1987 HIV	1988 AIDS	1992 AIDS	t_p	1981–1987 HIV	1988 AIDS	1992 AIDS	t_p
$\frac{1}{2}$ CDC	current 1987	30911	805	1018	3.99	23325	703	735	3.17	49833	987	3413	10.51
CDC		15604	809	1031	4.02	11745	708	737	3.29	24806	985	3538	11.81
Weibull		10229	791	967	4.08	7752	671	683	3.38	16727	1023	3398	9.82
$\frac{1}{2}$ CDC	earlier 1987	58457	1166	2973	6.75	39217	966	1306	4.31	92418	1527	17928	α
CDC		29851	1178	3172	7.03	19406	956	1300	4.31	46308	1519	18610	α
Weibull		19323	1176	3071	7.07	13006	954	1276	4.43	29425	1550	20322	α
$\frac{1}{2}$ CDC	current 1988	29617	786	969	3.90	24444	733	763	3.32	36854	840	1514	5.31
CDC		15106	792	994	3.95	12221	729	764	3.35	18401	833	1548	5.45
Weibull		10229	791	967	4.08	8580	719	770	3.59	12130	832	1447	5.46

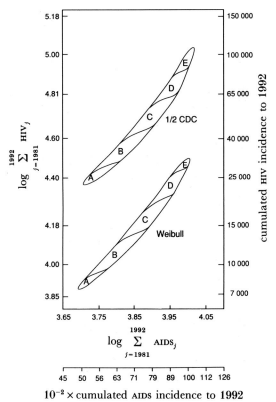

FIGURE 1. HIV incidence versus AIDS incidence: cumulated 1981–1992. Peak HIV incidence, pre 1984, A; 1984, B; 1985, C; after 1986, E.

TABLE 6. PREDICTED NEW AIDS CASES IN 1992: AS A FUNCTION OF PEAK ANNUAL HIV INCIDENCE DATE

(AIDS cases: current estimates for 1987.)

| incubation distribution | time period in which incidence of HIV infection peaks | | | | | | |
	1984	1985	1986	1987	1988	1989	1990
	lower ⎫ upper ⎭ bound of predicted AIDS cases in 1992						
$\frac{1}{2}$ CDC	735	958	1355	1707	2112	2369	2698
	1087	1578	2153	2508	2928	3176	3389
CDC	737	952	1353	1754	2078	2412	2658
	1095	1627	2131	2604	2927	3147	3478
Weibull	672	867	1241	1649	2030	2380	2942
	992	1432	2026	2427	2797	3109	3398

as it is at the start of 1989 (on which the predictions of table 4 were based) and as it might be at the start of 1990. In early 1988, linear exponential extrapolation of the epidemic was still plausible, generating the estimates of AIDS diagnoses up to the end of 1987 as in column 1 of table 2. Predictions based on these estimates using Weibull, CDC and half-CDC models are given in table 5. They are markedly different from the predictions based on our 'current' estimates to the end of 1987.

In early 1990, we might expect the estimated number of AIDS diagnoses in 1988 to be 777

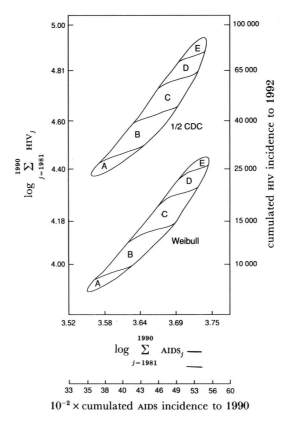

FIGURE 2. HIV incidence versus AIDS incidence: cumulated 1981–1990. Peak HIV incidence,
pre 1984, A; 1984, B; 1985, C; 1986, D; after 1986, E.

TABLE 7. YEARLY NUMBER OF NEW HIV INFECTIONS: BY DIFFERENT PEAK
ANNUAL HIV INCIDENCE DATE

(AIDS cases: current estimates for 1987; assumed incubation distribution: CDC rates.)

peak annual HIV incidence date: Jan. 1981 + t_p where $t_p \approx$

year	3.5	4.5	5.5	6.5	7.5	8.5	9.5
1981	364	493	595	541	592	643	670
1982	1349	1259	1211	1149	1145	1163	1176
1983	2960	2460	2106	2130	2001	1945	1933
1984	3846	3675	3125	3441	3158	3004	2975
1985	2962	4201	3959	4847	4505	4286	4285
1986	1351	3673	4282	5954	5808	5651	5777
1987	364	2457	3954	6377	6766	6882	7291
1988	58	1257	3116	5956	7122	7743	8614
1989	5	491	2097	4851	6775	8049	9526
1990	0	147	1205	3445	5824	7729	9861
1991	0	34	591	2133	4524	6857	9556
1992	0	6	247	1152	3176	5620	8669
$a\exp(bt+ct^2)$							
a	128	258	378	338	398	453	483
b	1.9638	1.248	0.8870	0.9063	0.7702	0.6791	0.6343
c	−0.2805	−0.1387	−0.0807	−0.0697	−0.0513	−0.0400	−0.0333

(table 2, column 2). Comparing predictions based on the 'best' estimates up to 1988 with those based on the 'current' estimates up to 1987, we can see a major reduction in the range, particularly at the upper end. (The predictions based on the best fitting model are virtually the same, because the 1988 estimate is close to the best fitting model using data up to 1987.) The main difference is that with the putative 1988 diagnoses, the peak in the epidemic of HIV infection can have occurred no later than mid-1986 ($t_p = 5.5$), whereas using only current 1987 data the peak could have occurred after 1988 i.e. new infections continually increasing in the period 1981 to 1988.

4. DISCUSSION

The results of this analysis illustrate three points. First, that for predictions of AIDS cases four to five years into the future, the back projection method is largely insensitive to the assumption one makes for the incubation period distribution. The two extreme distributions considered represent the fast and slow extremes of incubation period distribution usually proposed; distributions that lie between these two give predictions within the range of predictions that the two generate. The estimated number of new HIV infections, however, is highly sensitive to the assumed incubation period distribution; prediction of AIDS cases in the long term will be similarly sensitive.

Second, that each prediction of AIDS cases within the range of consistent predictions corresponds to a particular form for the HIV epidemic. This correspondence enables one to use a variety of data, of varying degrees of reliability and direct relevance, to assess the plausibility of each prediction. This use of additional data is a major attraction of the back projection method, which would otherwise be just another form of extrapolation. Assuming a form for the HIV epidemic and for the incubation period distribution is equivalent to assuming a certain form for the yearly number of AIDS cases. Unless further information is used, the back projection method would be equivalent to straightforward extrapolation of the AIDS cases. In this straightforward extrapolation, however, there is no way to incorporate accumulating information on the incubation period, changing levels of transmission and rates of HIV infection. Dissection of the extrapolation process in the back projection method focuses attention on where this extra information can be used.

Third, that the AIDS reports in 1988 have made a major impact on short and medium term projections. The range of predictions is much narrower, and considerably lower, than it was based on data available at the start of 1988. Preliminary estimates for 1988 diagnoses, based on 1988 reports, would generate a range of only two fold for 1992 predictions, compared to the 15-fold range based on data to the end of 1987.

The functional form used for the evolving HIV epidemic covers, at least approximately, the plausible models of the epidemic up to the present. It is clear, however, that models that give a peak between 1985 and 1987, consistent with available information on changing homosexual behaviour, predict implausibly low numbers of HIV infecteds in the years 1989–92 (see table 7). However, even if one allowed the yearly number of HIV infecteds to plateau at, say, the 1987 level, few extra AIDS cases would be generated by 1992. Thus in table 5, the best fitting and low predictions should perhaps be increased by 100 to 150. One might also, as in the Cox report, add an extra 20% for underreporting. Even so, this would bring the best estimate of new AIDS cases in 1992 to at most 1500, and the upper bound on predictions to about 4200; if one limits the range to those consistent with the available data on HIV transmission and the number of HIV infecteds, then an upper bound of some 3000 looks appropriate. This range of uncertainty will be greatly reduced if the 1989 data follow current trends. By the end of 1989, the range of predictions for 1992 may well be approximately 1000–2000.

REFERENCES

Brookmeyer, R. & Davison, A. 1989 Statistical methods for short term projections of AIDS incidence. *Statist. Med.* **8**, 23–34.

Department of Health Working Group 1988 Short term predictions of HIV infection and AIDS in England and Wales. London: HMSO.

Cox, D. R. 1988 Some remarks on the analysis of reporting delays. Appendix 8 of Department of Health Working Group Report.

Healy, M. J. R. 1988 Extrapolation forecasting. Appendix 6 of the Department of Health Working Group Report.

Johnson, A. M. & Gill, O. N. 1988 Evidence for recent changes in sexual behaviour in homosexual men in England and Wales. Appendix 5 of the Department of Health Working Group Report.

Zeger, S. L., See, L. C. & Diggle, P. J. 1989 Statistical methods for monitoring the AIDS epidemic. *Statist. Med.* **8**, 3–21.

Phil. Trans. R. Soc. Lond. B **325**, 135–145 (1989)   [**135**]

Printed in Great Britain

A PROCESS OF EVENTS WITH NOTIFICATION DELAY AND THE FORECASTING OF AIDS

By D. R. COX, F.R.S.[1], and G. F. MEDLEY[2]

[1] *Nuffield College, Oxford OX1 1NF, U.K.*

[2] *Department of Pure and Applied Biology, Imperial College of Science and Technology, London SW7 2BZ, U.K.*

Analysis and prediction of a point process are studied when there is delay in notifying the occurrence of events. A primarily parametric approach is taken to studying the rate of the underlying process and to predicting future properties of the system. Data on AIDS are used in illustration.

1. Introduction

This investigation was motivated by the need for short-term prediction of the AIDS epidemic (Healy & Tillett 1988). Brookmeyer & Damanio (1988) and Downs *et al.* (1987) have also considered this problem. The account here is, however, in a rather more general setting. Further details of the application are given in Cox, Working Group Report (1988).

Consider a point process of events occurring in continuous time in a Poisson process of rate $\lambda(t)$. When we wish to emphasize that $\lambda(t)$ depends on unknown parameters we write $\lambda(t;\rho)$. With a point at time t_i is associated a notification lag x_i; that is, the point is not entered into the data until time $t_i + x_i$, when both t_i and x_i are recorded. We treat the x_i as independent and identically distributed copies of a random variable X, having probability density function $f_X(x;\theta)$, depending on unknown parameters θ. In particular X_i is independent of T_i.

We consider two problems associated with this system. Suppose that the system is observed, either for $(-\infty, t_0)$ or for $(0, t_0)$. In the former case, all events occurring and notified before t_0 are available for analysis. In the second case only events occurring after the time origin are recorded; note the alternative possibility that events notified after the time origin are recorded regardless of the time of occurrence of the originating event.

In the first problem it is required to study the form of the rate function $\lambda(t)$. In the second problem there may be further properties (durations or costs, for instance) associated with the point events and it is required to predict some aspect of these at a future time, $v > t_0$.

In the application to AIDS that we have in mind, namely the short-term forecasting of the AIDS epidemic in the U.K., the point events are defined by patients newly diagnosed as having AIDS. The corresponding rate $\lambda(t)$ is currently increasing less than exponentially with t. The notification lag here is the delay between the diagnosis of a case and its notification to the Communicable Disease Surveillance Centre (CDSC), Public Health Laboratories. At present this lag is between a few weeks and, in extreme cases, 2 or more years. In the forecasting aspects of the problem we might be interested, for example, in the number of patients with AIDS alive at time v or in the number of patients with AIDS in hospital at time v. We shall see in §3 how these and similar features can be studied in the present framework. A quite different interpretation with a different focus of interest is obtained by identifying originating points with instants of infection and the delay with incubation period (Medley *et al.* 1988).

The main idealizations in the present formulation, again as regards AIDS, are that the process is formulated in continuous time, whereas data become available monthly; that there may be changes with time in the distribution of the delay X, and that there are some dependencies between the delays for different patients arising when collection centres submit their notifications in batches. The analysis could be extended to deal with these complications, but we have not done so.

2. ANALYSIS

Under the above assumptions if the process is observed for a time interval $A(t_0)$ ending at time t_0 and diagnosis–lag pairs $(t_1, x_1), \ldots, (t_n, x_n)$ are observed, the log likelihood is

$$\sum \log \lambda(t_i; \rho) + \sum \log f_X(x_i; \theta) - \int_{A(t_0)} \lambda(w; \rho) F_X(t_0 - w; \theta) \, \mathrm{d}w. \tag{1}$$

Note that, as explained in §1, when $A(t_0)$ is finite, the lower limit of the integral is determined in our formulation by the instance of occurrence of the originating event.

The integral will in general have to be evaluated repeatedly and so there is some gain in having parametric forms for which the integral can be found in closed form. In some of the discussion below we shall take the form of the rate function to be determined by semi-theoretical considerations, but for cautious empirical investigation a natural starting point for detecting departures from exponential form is

$$\lambda(t; \rho) = \exp{(\rho_0 + \rho_1 t - \rho_2 t^2)} = \exp{[\gamma_0 + \gamma_1(t_0 - t) - \gamma_2(t_0 - t)^2]}. \tag{2}$$

We have taken the negative sign for the quadratic term so that slowing down of an initial exponential growth is represented by $\rho_2 = \gamma_2 > 0$. The reparameterization in the second form has some advantages for computation, but suffers from the obvious disadvantage that the parameters change as t_0 changes.

Note that subject to the convergence of the integral involved, the likelihood is such that (1) associated with (2) would form a full exponential family were the lag distribution known.

Important special cases have (i) $\rho_1 = \rho_2 = 0$ and (ii) $\rho_2 = 0$. Null hypotheses corresponding to (i) and (ii) can be tested via the additional parameters in the usual way.

Although (2) is the natural starting point for testing exponentiality of growth, if departures are found it is important for prediction to consider rate functions broadly consistent with theoretical knowledge (Anderson et al. 1986; Isham 1988). We have fitted to the AIDS data not only (1) and (2) but a logistic function and, more importantly, a linear logistic function that is initially exponential switching gradually to a linear phase. It corresponds approximately to one of the more realistic models considered by Isham (1988). Of course, the linear phase will itself be of limited duration.

Now the distribution of X will often be of small intrinsic interest, it being a 'nuisance' preventing direct observation of the instants of diagnosis and it will then be sensible to choose a parametric form on the basis of mathematical convenience, or to proceed non-parametrically. Simple forms that link well with (2) are (a) an exponential distribution, $\theta \, \mathrm{e}^{-\theta x}$; (b) a linear combination of exponentials, or more generally, a density with a rational Laplace transform, thus including gamma distributions of integer index and mixtures thereof, for example a mixture of two gamma distributions of index one,

$$\theta_0 \, \theta_1^2 \, x \, \mathrm{e}^{-\theta_1 x} + (1 - \theta_0) \, \theta_2^2 \, x \, \mathrm{e}^{-\theta_2 x}; \tag{3}$$

(c) the cumulative distribution function

$$1 - \exp\left(-\theta_1 x - \theta_2 x^2\right). \tag{4}$$

Here we require both component parameters to be non-negative and at least one to be strictly positive.

In all these cases the log likelihood (1) is available in closed form. We shall not give every possibility in detail but the following special cases are worth noting.

First if $A(t_0) = (-\infty, t_0)$ and $\lambda(t;\rho) = \exp(\rho_0 + \rho_1 t)$, with $\rho_1 > 0$, then the integral in (1) is

$$\rho_1^{-1} \exp\left(\rho_0 + \rho_1 t_0\right) E\left(e^{-\rho_1 X}; \theta\right), \tag{5}$$

i.e. it is expressible in terms of the moment generating function of X and so, in particular, is available in simple form for distributions with rational Laplace transforms. If, however, $A(t_0) = (0, t_0)$, the form typically necessary whenever there have been many points before the start of recording, then the integral takes the more complicated form

$$\exp\left(\rho_0 + \rho_1 t_0\right) \int_0^{t_0} e^{-\rho_1 z} F_X(z)\, \mathrm{d}z;$$

this can also be evaluated explicitly in important cases.

In the special case in which $A(t_0) = (-\infty, t_0)$, $\rho_1 > 0$ and $F_X(x;\theta) = 1 - e^{-\theta x}$ the log likelihood (1) can be written in the canonical exponential family form

$$\psi_0 n + \psi_1 \sum t_i + \psi_2\left(-\sum x_i\right) - \exp\left(\psi_0 + \psi_1 t_0\right)\left[\psi_1(\psi_1 + \psi_2)\right]^{-1}, \tag{6}$$

where
$$\psi_0 = \rho_0 + \log\theta, \psi_1 = \rho_1, \psi_2 = \theta.$$

It follows in particular from this that the simple estimate of the mean reporting lag, $\sum x_1/n$, has expectation approximately $(\theta + \rho_1)^{-1}$ rather than θ^{-1} and so is seriously biased unless ρ_1 is small compared with θ. Such biases are likely to arise much more generally if aspects of the distribution of X are estimated directly from the reported lags, unless either the lags are nearly all small compared with ρ_1^{-1} or values near the end of the data are discarded. Of course, the full likelihood analysis automatically corrects for such biases. Some further aspects of the study of reporting delays are discussed in §5.

The form of rate function of considerable interest in connection with AIDS, especially for testing for exponential form, is probably (2) with $\rho_1 > 0$ and $\rho_2 \geqslant 0$. If we take the interval of observation to be $(-\infty, t_0)$ and the distribution of X to be either (4) or a combination of exponentials, the integral in the log likelihood can be evaluated explicitly. For the interval $(0, t_0)$ the results are slightly more complicated, but for $\rho_2 > 0$, the answer is expressed in terms of Dawson's function

$$D(x) = \exp\left(-\tfrac{1}{2}x^2\right) \int_0^x \exp\left(\tfrac{1}{2}t^2\right) \mathrm{d}t. \tag{7}$$

We give the detailed result only for a single exponential and $\rho_2 > 0$, when the integral becomes

$$\theta\pi^{\frac{1}{2}}\rho_2^{-\frac{1}{2}} \exp\left[\rho_0 + \tfrac{1}{4}(\rho_1 + \theta)^2 \rho_2^{-1}\right] \Phi\left[(2\rho_2)^{\frac{1}{2}}t_0 - (\rho_1 + \theta)(2\rho_2^{-\frac{1}{2}})\right] \tag{8}$$

where $\Phi(x)$ is the standardized normal integral.

From whichever of these expressions is appropriate maximum likelihood estimates, their asymptotic covariance matrix, likelihood ratio statistics and profile log likelihood functions for individual component parameters can be found. It is possible also to develop simple score tests for null hypotheses such as $\rho_2 = 0$ or $\rho_1 = 0$, assuming that $\rho_2 = 0$, or $\rho_1 = \rho_2 = 0$, but we have preferred to study parameters via their profile log likelihoods, despite the extra computation involved. Adequacy of a model can be tested either by comparing observed and fitted numbers of events in suitable time intervals, or by fitting expanded models in the usual way.

3. PREDICTION

We now turn to methods for predicting future properties of the system analysed above. Errors of forecasting will be of three types, namely errors arising from the random system as formulated, errors in estimating the parameters in the model and errors arising from misspecification of the process. In many applications, and certainly in the application to AIDS, the last of these three sources is the most important, even in quite short-term forecasting.

Suppose that attached to each point event is a random function of time, independent and identically distributed from event to event and independent of the point process. For an event at t, i.e. a case diagnosed at t, denote the function by $I(t;v)$ and consider the total at time v of these functions associated with all points occurring up to v, i.e. let

$$Y(v) = \int_{-\infty}^{v} I(t;v)\, \mathrm{d}N(t), \tag{9}$$

where $N(t)$ is the counting function of the originating point process, i.e. the number of points occurring at or before time t. Note that we are estimating actual events and not just notified events. If, for instance, attached to each point is a random survival time, then $I(t;v)$ is one during the survival time of the point and zero otherwise and $Y(v)$ is the number of individual points alive at time v. There is, however, no need to restrict I to be a binary indicator function.

The limits of integration in (9) are appropriate when the function of interest is zero before the originating point, and this will be the case in our applications, but there is no difficulty in dealing with 'two-sided' functions of interest, in fact by taking the integral in (9) to be over $(-\infty, \infty)$.

The main properties of $Y(v)$ follow from Campbell's theorem (Cox & Miller 1965, chapter 9); note that a version for nonstationary point processes is required and that the assumption that the originating point process is a Poisson process could easily be relaxed. The key results are as follows.

For binary I, $Y(v)$ has a Poisson distribution and under the independence assumptions set out above

$$E[Y(c)] = \int_{-\infty}^{v} E[I(t;v)]\, \lambda(t;\rho)\, \mathrm{d}t. \tag{10}$$

Generally if the number of points contributing to $Y(v)$ is large, it follows from the central limit theorem that the process $[Y(v)]$ is approximately a nonstationary Gaussian process with the above mean and with

$$\mathrm{cov}\,[Y(v_1), Y(v_2)] = \int_{-\infty}^{\min(v_1, v_2)} E[I(t;v_1)\, I(t;v_2)]\, \lambda(t;\rho)\, \mathrm{d}t. \tag{11}$$

Thus if $I(t;v)$ indicates whether a point originating at t is still alive at time v, then

$$E[I(t;v)] = \mathscr{F}_S(v-t;\phi),$$

[100]

where $\mathscr{F}_S(s;\phi)$ is the survivor function attached to each point, assumed to depend on an unknown parameter ϕ.

Now to predict $Y(v)$ on the basis of observations up to time t_0, in a non-Bayesian treatment we first find the conditional distribution of $Y(v)$ given the data and supposing the unknown parameters governing the process to be known. Then we insert efficient estimates of the unknown parameters. Finally, in principle at least, we adjust the resulting prediction intervals for the estimation errors in the unknown parameters. In practice the last step is often omitted as a minor refinement and sometimes the first step is replaced by an approximation using the 'best' linear predictor and the associated standard deviation. In the Bayesian treatment the posterior distribution of $Y(v)$ is computed directly in a standard way.

In the present situation $Y(v)$ is the sum of three independent terms corresponding to

(a) those points already observed, i.e. occurring and notified before t_0;

(b) those points occurring before t_0 but not notified;

(c) those points occurring in the interval (t_0, v).

We treat in more detail the case corresponding to survival times although the argument generalizes fairly easily. Then contributions (b) and (c) have Poisson distributions with means respectively

$$\left.\begin{array}{c} \displaystyle\int_{-\infty}^{t_0} \lambda(t;\rho)\,\mathscr{F}_S(v-t,\phi)\,\mathscr{F}_X(t_0-t;\theta)\,\mathrm{d}t, \\[3ex] \displaystyle\int_{t_0}^{v} \lambda(t;\rho)\,\mathscr{F}_S(v-t;\phi)\,\mathrm{d}t, \end{array}\right\} \tag{12}$$

whereas (a) is a sum of independent binary contributions from those individual points occurring and notified before t_0 and known to be still 'alive' at t_0. Provided that notification of death is virtually immediate, the contribution of one such point occurring at t_i, say, and still 'alive' at t_0 has expectation

$$\mathscr{F}_S(v-t_i)/\mathscr{F}_S(t_0-t_i) \tag{13}$$

so that the total contribution has expectation the sum of (13) over all recorded points still 'alive' at t_0. It will often be a reasonable conservative approximation to treat the corresponding distribution to be of Poisson form and hence to conclude that $Y(v)$ has a Poisson distribution with mean, $\mu(v, t_0; \rho, \theta, \phi)$, the sum of the three contributions just specified. If there is a time delay between death and notification, then (13) needs modification.

In one of the simpler special cases in which

$$\lambda(t;\rho) = \exp(\rho_0 + \rho_1 t),\, \mathscr{F}_X(x;\theta) = \mathrm{e}^{-\theta x},\, \mathscr{F}_S(s;\phi) = \mathrm{e}^{-s\phi} \tag{14}$$

the resulting Poisson mean is

$$r(t_0) \exp[-\phi(v-t_0)] + \exp(\rho_0 + \rho_1 v)/(\rho_1 + \phi)$$
$$- \theta \exp[\rho_0 + \rho_1 t_0 - \phi(v-t_0)]/[(\rho_1 + \phi)(\rho_1 + \theta + \phi)], \quad (15)$$

where $r(t_0)$ is the number of points notified before t_0 and still 'alive' at t_0. Note that in this particular case, the contribution (a) has a binomial distribution of index $r(t_0)$.

We thus obtain Poisson prediction limits on $Y(v)$ on replacing the parameters by maximum likelihood estimates.

Note finally that if Y is a variable to be predicted having a Poisson distribution with large mean μ and if μ is estimated by m having standard error s, then approximate prediction limits for Y are

$$m \pm k_\alpha (m + s^2)^{\frac{1}{2}}, \tag{16}$$

where k_α is the appropriate normal multiplier. Of course, as noted above, in many situations errors in specifying the model, in particular the form of the rate function $\lambda(t; \rho)$, are likely to predominate.

4. APPLICATION TO AIDS

In this section we apply the above to short-term prediction of the total numbers of AIDS cases diagnosed in the United Kingdom. The number of AIDS cases diagnosed and still living is also of considerable interest and can be tackled by the arguments of section 3, but we defer discussion of this.

The AIDS notification data were supplied by the CDSC for all cases up to 1 July 1988. A fairly detailed description of the data and some important *caveats* can be found elsewhere (Cox, Working Group Report 1988; Healy & Tillett 1988; Tillett *et al.* 1988). For each case the calendar months of diagnosis and of the arrival of the report to CDSC were given. We excluded those cases that were known to be visitors to the U.K. from abroad, and those cases with an incomplete date of diagnosis (the date of report is always complete). Thus we used 1470 out of the 1598 available cases. Our final predictions are divided by 1470/1532 to take account of those cases that are not included in the full analysis owing to incomplete data, but who were not visitors. Where necessary the originating event was chosen to be 1 January 1979. The diagnoses were assumed to have been made in the middle of each month, thus half a month was subtracted from the time of diagnosis and from t_0 (1 July 1988).

We have investigated the fit of the exponential model by taking (2) as an empirical incidence function, and testing the hypothesis that $\rho_2 = 0$. We used many different distributions for the reporting lag, and give the results from one here, namely the weighted sum of two first order gamma distributions. Years are the time units used throughout. The improvement in log likelihood by including ρ_2 is 18.54. The profile log likelihood function for ρ_2 is roughly quadratic with a slight skewness towards higher values, thus indicating that the epidemic is not described adequately by simple exponential growth. Healy & Tillett (1988) reached the same conclusion about ρ_2 using least squares methods.

To obtain a reasonable approximation to the lag distribution, it was necessary to take account of the discreteness of the recorded data at lags of 0, 1 and 2 months. The dates are recorded as calendar months, thus a lag of 0 months includes 0 to 30 days, 1 month includes 1 to 61 days and so on. The lag distribution is altered so that for month $n (= 0, 1, 2)$

$$p(n) = \int [\theta_0 \theta_1^2 x e^{-\theta_1 x} + (1 - \theta_0) \theta_2^2 x e^{-\theta_2 x}] \, dx,$$

where the integral is over the appropriate month.

A very long tail in the delay distribution would be unobservable, and yet would inflate the estimated number of diagnoses. We have arbitrarily supposed that the chance of a delay of more than 3 years is negligible, and deleted lags greater than this from the likelihood (six observations). Figure 1 compares the observed lag distribution for all 133 cases diagnosed before 1985 with that calculated from the distribution in table 1.

Epidemiological theory predicts the initial exponential increase in the number of cases, and

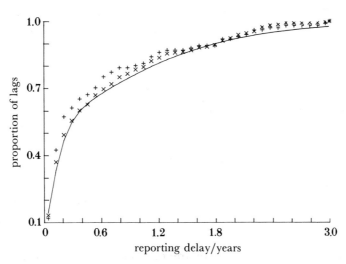

FIGURE 1. Comparison of observed frequency distribution by month of reporting lags with fitted distribution. The plus signs (+) are observed data reported up to June 1988 and diagnosed prior to 1985 (excluding visitors and lags greater than 3 years, $n = 101$). The crosses (×) are observed data reported up to June 1988 and diagnosed before 1986 ($n = 264$). The line is a mixture of two first order gamma distributions fitted with the linear–logistic incidence function (see table 1). The early cases were chosen to minimize bias towards shorter lags in observed reporting distribution, but may not be an accurate representation of the true, prevailing distribution.

TABLE 1. LOG LIKELIHOOD ESTIMATES AND VALUES, ℓ, FOR DIFFERENT INCIDENCE FUNCTIONS AND REPORTING LAG OF A MIXTURE OF TWO FIRST ORDER GAMMA DISTRIBUTIONS (3)

ρ_1	ρ_2	ρ_3	ρ_4	θ_1	θ_2	θ_3	ℓ
quadratic exponential (equation 2)							
−2.57	1.55	0.052 32	—	0.57	10.65	1.52	5353.58
logistic (equation 17)							
8.22	0.97	1519	—	0.57	11.36	1.49	5348.09
linear–logistic (equation 18)							
70.99	162.06	13.57	0.82	0.57	11.35	1.52	5350.80

also forecasts that as the epidemic progresses, 'exponential' ceases to be an adequate description of the data and the 'next approximation' is required (Anderson *et al.* 1986). To this end we considered the logistic and the linear–logistic equations:

$$\lambda(t;\rho) = \rho_3/[1 + \exp(\rho_1 - \rho_2 t)], \tag{17}$$

$$\lambda(t;\rho) = (\rho_1 + \rho_2 t)/[1 + \rho_3 \rho_1 \exp(-\rho_4 t)]. \tag{18}$$

Over the period of the data, there is no great difference between the incidence functions, and the maximum log likelihoods are not greatly different. Table 1 gives the estimated parameter values and maximum log likelihoods, and table 2 shows the predictions calculated from them.

It is possible to estimate confidence intervals for the predictions derived from the logistic model (17) by setting

$$\rho_2 = P\bigg/\int\!\!\int_B \lambda(t;\rho)\,\mathcal{F}_S(s;\theta)\,\mathrm{d}s\,\mathrm{d}t$$

where B is the time region over which the prediction is being made, and P is the prediction. Essentially, the particular form of the logistic equation allows us to substitute parameter P for

[103]

TABLE 2. COMPARISON BETWEEN PREDICTIONS OF THREE INCIDENCE FUNCTIONS[a]

year quarter	observed notifications	notifications			diagnoses		
		quad. exp.	logistic	linear logistic	quad. exp.	logistic	linear logistic
1987 1	134	121	123	123	162	167	164
2	132	141	143	142	187	190	188
3	175	162	164	163	213	214	213
4	147	186	185	186	241	238	239
1988 1	186	211	207	209	271	260	264
2	153	237	228	232	302	281	290
3	196	265	248	256	333	300	315
4	188	294	266	280	365	316	339
1989 1	—	324	284	303	397	331	362
2	—	354	300	326	428	343	384
3	—	383	314	348	458	353	405
4	—	412	326	370	485	361	425
1990 1	—	439	337	390	510	368	443
2	—	465	347	410	532	374	461
3	—	488	355	429	551	378	477
4	—	509	362	447	565	382	493
1991 1	—	526	368	464	575	385	508
2	—	540	373	480	581	387	522
3	—	550	377	496	582	389	536
4	—	555	380	511	578	390	549
1992 1	—	557	383	525	569	392	562
2	—	555	386	539	556	392	574
3	—	548	388	552	539	393	586
4	—	537	389	565	518	394	598

[a] Note that figures beyond the second quarter of 1988 are predictions. The number of notifications received by CDSC are given for comparison. These figures differ slightly from those published previously (Working Group 1988) because they include Scotland, i.e. the predictions are for the U.K.

ρ_2, and obtain a confidence interval for P in the usual manner. Generally the confidence interval is asymmetric, with the upper bound being further from the point estimate than the lower bound.

Approximate confidence intervals for other incidence functions can be obtained by computing the log likelihood for a grid of values in parameter space. When plotted as in figure 2, the confidence interval can be fitted by eye. We chose to fix the lag distribution at the point estimate value, and to only vary the incidence parameters, ρ.

This was partly to reduce the computing resources required and partly because the lag distribution compared well with observation (figure 1). The effects of ρ on both the likelihood and predictions are non-linear and highly correlated. It should be possible to transform the parameters and to choose combinations of them that make their effect on the log likelihood linear and orthogonal, and thus reduce the computation involved greatly.

Table 2 shows predictions of numbers of diagnoses and notifications for the three functions for quarter years to 1992. The differences between the forecasts are major, even after a year or so. The logistic curve moves relatively quickly to an asymptote after departing from simple exponential growth; this is unrealistic in view of the heterogeneity in progression from infection to disease in individual patients. The quadratic exponential is valuable to represent small perturbations from simple exponential growth, but the fact that it peaks relatively rapidly and

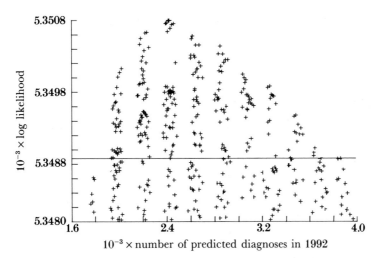

FIGURE 2. The log likelihood values for different combinations of ρ_1, ρ_2, ρ_3 and ρ_4 assuming a linear–logistic incidence (18) and a fixed lag distribution (see table 1). The number of diagnoses expected throughout 1992 is calculated from ρ. Because the effects of ρ on both the likelihood and predictions are nonlinear and highly correlated, many more evaluations were calculated than shown on the figure.

then declines symmetrically is also unrealistic in the present context. The linear–logistic model is the most plausible choice due to theoretical justification.

The major source of variability is the choice of incidence function. The present predictions are at best reasonably accurate for homosexual men for perhaps three years ahead; information on other risk groups (intra-venous drug users, for example) is too scanty for separate prediction to be sensible.

5. DISTRIBUTION OF REPORTING DELAYS

We now consider briefly some further aspects of the study of reporting delays. In the previous part of the paper these have been studied indirectly via maximum likelihood fitting of a composite model. Suppose, however, we wish to study the delays directly, preferably by some simpler method, and in particular to examine stability of the distribution in time.

Suppose as before that events corresponding here to diagnoses, occur in a Poisson process of rate $\lambda(t)$. To each event is attached a reporting delay, X, having a distribution with density $f_x(x)$ and cumulative distribution function $F_X(x)$. Observations are made over the period $(-\infty, t_0)$. The distribution of delay for individuals observed to be diagnosed (near) t has the truncated distribution $f_X(x)/F_X(t_0-t)$ for $0 \leqslant x \leqslant t_0-t$. Therefore, to examine the constancy of the distribution in time a simple procedure is to truncate all delay times at some suitable x', omitting all diagnoses after t_0-x'. The resulting delay times sorted by time of diagnosis should then have a fixed distribution. Clearly this gives us no information about the delays longer than x'.

If however, individuals are sorted by time s of report and the corresponding distributions of delay examined, biases arise. If T, S, X are random variables representing time of diagnosis, report and delay, then the conditional distribution of X given $S = s$ is

$$f_X(x)\,\lambda(s-x) \bigg/ \int_0^\infty f_X(u)\,\lambda(s-u)\,\mathrm{d}u.$$

[105]

Now this is equal to $f_X(x)$ for all x, s if and only if the rate $\lambda(.)$ is constant. In particular if $\lambda(t) = \alpha e^{\beta t}$, the conditional density is, for all s,

$$f_X(x) e^{-\beta x} \int_0^\infty f_X(u) e^{-\beta u} du.$$

Thus if $\beta > 0$, the bias is in favour of the shorter times, the conditional distribution being independent of s, i.e. showing no trend in time. Note, however, that if the epidemic grows subexponentially, so that in effect β is slowly decreasing with s, the conditional distribution of X given time of report, s, shows increasing delays as s increases. This is a consequence of the 'biased' sampling. More generally, the conditional density is independent of s if and only if the rate is exponential.

To see this last point qualitatively, consider an idealized case in which half the delays are quite small and the other half long. If initially the epidemic grows rapidly, the conditional distribution of delay at a fixed time of report is strongly biased towards the short times. If now there is a switch to a constant rate, the conditional distribution has a transient phase and then tends to the 'true' distribution, i.e. delays will appear to have lengthened.

Plots of the distribution of delay time sorted by date of report show some tendency for delays to lengthen, as might be expected from the above discussion. If, on the other hand, the cases are sorted by quarter of diagnosis and delays over 8 months omitted, the mean delays are those in table 3.

TABLE 3. MEAN AND STANDARD DEVIATION OF DELAY DISTRIBUTION,
DELAYS TRUNCATED AT 8 MONTHS

	1986				1987			
quarter of diagnosis...	1	2	3	4	1	2	3	4
mean/months	3.02	2.81	2.43	3.03	2.74	2.19	2.14	2.03
s.d./months	2.38	2.36	2.32	2.41	2.31	2.13	2.27	1.97

There is some decrease in the shorter reporting delays in 1987: it is from the data alone impossible to separate changes in 1988 from changes in incidence and it is also effectively impossible to study the frequency and length of very long delays.

Although we shall not explore the matter in detail, it would be possible to fit a model in which the distribution of delays depends simply on the time of diagnosis. If, however, rather arbitrary dependence were allowed there is clearly some practical or total indeterminacy; any recent fall in numbers reported could be explained by a recent increase in reporting lags.

We are grateful to Dr V. Isham for very helpful comments. The data on case notifications was kindly supplied by CDSC.

REFERENCES

Anderson, R. M., Medley, G. F., May, R. M. & Johnson, A. E. 1986 A preliminary study of the transmission dynamics of the human immunodeficiency virus (HIV), the causative agent of AIDS. *IMA J. Math. appl. Med. Biol.* **3**, 229–263.
Brookmeyer, R. & Damiano, A. 1988 Statistical methods for short-term projections of AIDS incidence. *Stat. Med.* **8**, 5–20.
Cox, D. R. (chairman) Department of Health Working Group Report 1988 Short-term prediction of HIV infection and AIDS in England and Wales. London: HMSO.

Cox, D. R. & Isham, V. 1980 *Point processes*. London: Chapman & Hall.

Cox, D. R. & Miller, H. D. 1965 *Theory of stochastic processes*. London: Chapman & Hall.

Downs, A. M., Ancelle, R. M., Jager, J. C. & Brunet, J. B. 1987 AIDS in Europe; current trends and short-term predictions estimated from surveillance data, January 1981–June 1986. *AIDS* 1, 53–57.

Healy, M. J. R. & Tillett, H. E. 1988 Short-term extrapolation of the AIDS epidemic (with discussion). *Jl R. statist. Soc.* A 151, 50–61.

Isham, V. 1988 Mathematical modelling of the transmission dynamics of HIV infection and AIDS: a review. *Jl R. statist. Soc.* 151, 5–30.

Medley, G. F., Billard, L., Cox, D. R. & Anderson, R. M. 1988 The distribution of the incubation period for the acquired immunodeficiency syndrome (AIDS). *Proc. R. Soc. Lond.* B 233, 367–377.

Tillett, H. E., Galbraith, N. S., Overton, S. E. & Porter, K. 1988 Routine surveillance data on AIDS & HIV infections in the U.K.: a description of the data available and their use for short-term planning. *Epidem. Inf.* 100, 157–169.

Phil. Trans. R. Soc. Lond. B **325**, 147–151 (1989)   [**147**]

Printed in Great Britain

THE OVERALL DISTRIBUTION OF SURVIVAL
TIMES FOR U.K. AIDS PATIENTS

By GILLIAN K. REEVES

Department of Mathematics, Imperial College of Science and Technology, London SW7 2BZ, U.K.

Data on the survival times of 997 U.K. AIDS patients are analysed with the aim of deriving a simple form for the overall survival distribution. The exponential and Weibull distributions are modified to accommodate specific features of the data, in particular, the recording of survival times to the nearest month and the occurrence of a significant proportion of cases recorded as having zero time on study. The final model has a probability 0.08 of underlying survival time being zero and, given non-zero survival time, takes the form of an exponential distribution with mean of 14.95 months. The results are in close agreement with those of a study of New York City patients as well as the empirical data.

1. INTRODUCTION

The aim of this paper is to find a simple representation for the overall distribution of survival time (time from diagnosis to death) for U.K. AIDS patients. The data consist of information on the first 997 U.K. AIDS cases; that is, all cases reported to the Communicable Disease Surveillance Centre and the Communicable Diseases (Scotland) Unit by the end of September 1987. For an analysis of survival time as a dependent variable based on the same data see Overton *et al.* (1988). The data contain the following features.

A significant proportion of cases have survival times that are effectively zero (diagnosis and death virtually simultaneous). Fewer individuals have survival times that are relatively long. The study of short survival times is further complicated by the fact that recording was to the nearest month.

The first two points mean that models that allow for the possibility of subpopulations at a much greater or much lower risk than the remainder of the population need to be considered; this is a common requirement in survival analysis. The above issues were studied by the maximum likelihood fitting of models based on the commonly used exponential and Weibull distributions.

2. THE MODELS

2.1. *Modification of the basic exponential and Weibull distributions*

First, although some of the recorded zeros are accountable via the continuous distribution because of the rounding, it was found necessary to introduce a point concentration at zero into the basic continuous distributions; thus the new density function, $f'(t)$, and survivor function, $S'(t)$, are given by

$$f'(t) = \begin{cases} \theta & (t = 0), \\ (1-\theta)f(t) & (t > 0), \end{cases}$$

$$S'(t) = \begin{cases} (1-\theta) & (t = 0), \\ (1-\theta)S(t) & (t > 0), \end{cases}$$

[109]

where $f(t)$ and $S(t)$ denote the basic Weibull or exponential density function and survivor function, respectively and θ represents the probability of zero survival time.

To check whether the simple functional form accounts for long term survivors, we can examine models in which there is a non-zero probability, γ, of 'long-term' survival, i.e. in effect an atom of probability at infinity can be incorporated into the model. In this case, the density and survivor functions, respectively, are,

$$f''(t) = \begin{cases} \theta & (t = 0), \\ (1-\theta-\gamma)f(t) & (t > 0), \\ \gamma & (t = \infty), \end{cases}$$

$$S''(t) = \gamma + (1-\theta-\gamma)\,S(t),$$

where γ now denotes the probability of long term survival and $f(t)$ and $S(t)$ are simple parametric forms as before.

One further adjustment was made to all of the above models. Because all dates were recorded to the nearest month, it is necessary to distinguish between θ, the actual probability of zero survival time, and π_0, a function of θ, which represents the probability of being recorded as having zero survival time. For the present analysis it was assumed that the time of diagnosis was distributed uniformly over a month, in which case π_0 can be written as

$$\pi_0 = \int_0^1 [1 - S^*(1-t)]\,\mathrm{d}t = \int_0^1 [1 - S^*(u)]\,\mathrm{d}u,$$

where $S^*(t)$ is the survivor function associated with the particular model, so in the case of the single atom model $S^*(t) = S'(t)$ and similarly for the two atom model $S^*(t) = S''(t)$. If the time period involved had been more than a month, for example if dates were given only to the nearest quarter, then a more appropriate distribution for the time of diagnosis, say $g(t)$, might depend in some way on the rate of new cases in which case π_0 would be given by

$$\pi_0 = \int_0^1 g(t)\,[1 - S^*(1-t)]\,\mathrm{d}t = \int_0^1 g(1+u)\,[1 - S^*(u)]\,\mathrm{d}u.$$

Of course, similar versions of the above expression could be used for the probability of survival time j months $(j = 1, 2, \ldots)$ but were considered unnecessary in this case.

If the exponential distribution or Weibull distribution is adapted to incorporate this discreteness in the data as well as a single atom at zero the resulting log likelihood for a censored sample is

$$\ell = n_0 \log(\pi_0) + \sum_{i \in u} \log[f'(t_i)] + \sum_{i \in c} \log[S'(t_i)],$$

where n_0 denotes the number of patients with time on study recorded as zero, t_i denotes the recorded survival time for the ith individual, and the subgroups C and U refer to the sets of censored and uncensored individuals, respectively. The log likelihood for the two-atom model can be similarly obtained by substituting $f''(t)$ and $S''(t)$ for $f'(t)$ and $S'(t)$, respectively.

3. Application and conclusions

3.1. *Application*

Of the 997 cases discussed in §1, death dates were known for 678 cases; the last known alive date could be specified for 319 including 15 cases that were censored because they were lost to follow-up; all visitors from abroad were excluded from the analysis. The following models (designated (a)–(d)) discussed in §2, were fitted using NAG subroutines, the integral π_0 was evaluated numerically within each iteration of the maximization procedure.

(a) An exponential distribution supplemented by a probability, θ, of zero survival time.

(b) A Weibull distribution supplemented by a probability, θ, of zero survival time.

(c) An exponential distribution supplemented by a probability, θ, of zero survival time and by a probability, γ, of 'long-term' survival.

(d) A Weibull distribution supplemented by a probability, θ, of zero survival time and by a probability, γ, of 'long-term' survival.

3.2. *Conclusions*

The results are summarized in table 1. The estimates of the parameter γ in both models (c) and (d) were not only non-significant but also negligible in value indicating that the probability of surviving for a relatively long period of time is accounted for by the exponential or Weibull component.

TABLE 1. PARAMETER ESTIMATES AND SELECTED CONFIDENCE INTERVALS
FOR MODELS (a) AND $(b)^a$

model	$\hat{\lambda}$	$\hat{\kappa}$	$\hat{\theta}$	l_{max}
(a)				
2-parameter exponential	0.067		0.080	-2450.13
(95% c.i.)	[0.061, 0.073]		[0.061, 0.101]	
(b)				
3-parameter Weibull	0.067	1.018	0.082	-2450.04

^{a} θ, probability at zero; exponential, $S(t) = e^{-\lambda t}$; Weibull, $S(t) = e^{(-\lambda t)^\kappa}$.

From the results of the remaining single atom models (a) and (b) it is clear that the underlying distribution is very close to an exponential distribution as can be seen from the estimated index in the Weibull model, which is almost equal to unity. This is confirmed by the non-significance of the difference in maximized log-likelihoods corresponding to a X^2 statistic of only 0.1804. The parameter θ is of particular interest and in the case of the exponential model has a value of 0.0802; this implies that about 80 of the 110 cases recorded as having zero time on study were genuine zeros, the others being a direct result of the recording procedure.

Because of the possible asymmetry of the log-likelihoods for all of these models standard errors for the estimates were not calculated; instead, confidence intervals were obtained via the profile log-likelihoods (figures 1 and 2); these indicate that $\hat{\lambda}$, in particular, is quite well defined.

Apart from extending the model parametrically, another method for testing the 'goodness of fit' is to compare an empirical version of the survival curve with that obtained under the assumed model. In this case, not only is the difference in maximized log-likelihoods for the exponential and Weibull models non-significant but the fit to the empirical data (figure 3) is

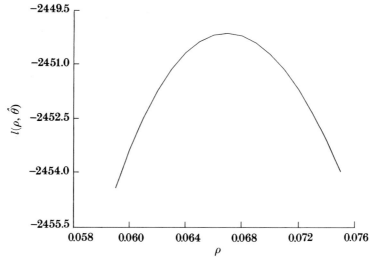

FIGURE 1. Profile log-likelihood for ρ.

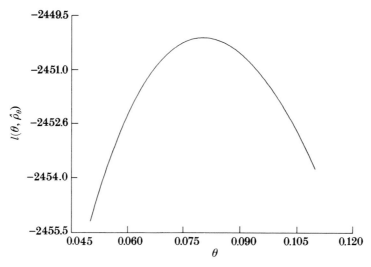

FIGURE 2. Profile log-likelihood for θ.

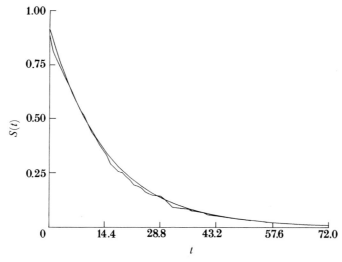

FIGURE 3. Fitted survivor function (smooth curve) and the Kaplan–Meier estimate (jagged curve); t, time/months.

excellent. Thus it appears that the very simple and convenient exponential model (*a*) is suitable for application. That is, we take a probability 0.080 of underlying survival time time being zero. Conditionally on non-zero survival time we take an exponential distribution with mean 14.950 months. Table 2 summarizes some properties.

TABLE 2. THE FITTED DISTRIBUTION

probability of zero survival time	0.080
probability of surviving at least	
1 month	0.860
3 months	0.753
6 months	0.616
12 months	0.412
24 months	0.185
36 months	0.083
median survival time/months	9.110
mean survival time/months	13.750

These results are in remarkably close agreement with those from a study of some 5833 New York City patients (Rothenberg *et al.* 1987). The number of New York City patients whose time on study was given as zero to the nearest day was 663; this constitutes about 11.37 % of all cases, which is close to the value of 11.03 % for the U.K. data. The median survival time for the New York City data, excluding cases with time on study recorded as zero, was 11.4 months compared with a corresponding value of 10.36 months under the exponential model for the U.K.

The contribution of reporting doctors who supplied the follow-up information and of Elizabeth Overton who prepared the data set is gratefully appreciated.

REFERENCES

Overton, S. E., Juritz, J. M., Gill, O. N., Kennedy, A. N., Wright, A. L. & Marasca, G. 1988 Survival analysis of the first 1000 cases of AIDS reported in the U.K. In *Proceedings of the 4th International Conference on AIDS, Stockholm* (poster no. 4593).

Rothenberg, R., Woelfe, M., Stoneburner, R., Milberg, J., Parker, R. & Truman, B. 1987 Survival with the acquired immunodeficiency syndrome. *New Engl. J. Med.* **317**, 1297–1302.

Phil. Trans. R. Soc. Lond. B **325**, 153–161 (1989) [153]

Printed in Great Britain

EVIDENCE FOR RECENT CHANGES IN SEXUAL BEHAVIOUR IN HOMOSEXUAL MEN IN ENGLAND AND WALES

By A. M. JOHNSON[1] and O. N. GILL[2]

[1] *Academic Department of Genito-Urinary Medicine, University College and Middlesex School of Medicine, The Middlesex Hospital, London W1N 8AA, U.K.*

[2] *PHLS Communicable Disease Surveillance Centre, 61 Colindale Avenue, London NW9 5EQ, U.K.*

Over 80% of cases of Acquired Immune Deficiency Syndrome (AIDS) in England and Wales have occurred in homosexual men. Changes in sexual behaviour in this group may have a substantial influence on the incidence of Human Immunodeficiency Virus (HIV) infection and will therefore be crucial in determining future cases of AIDS.

This paper critically weighs the indirect and direct evidence for changes in behaviour in homosexual men since the advent of the AIDS epidemic. The paper reports on falling incidence of gonorrhoea, hepatitis B and syphilis in homosexual men, the changes being most marked from 1985 onwards. Data on temporal trends in HIV prevalence and incidence in homosexual men are reviewed. These suggest that the maximum incidence of HIV infection occurred in 1982–84 and may have fallen since then.

Evidence for a concomitant change in sexual behaviour is reported from several sources. This points towards a recent change in sexual behaviour characterized by reduction in the numbers of partners and adoption of safer sexual practices. In some places change may have occurred as early as 1983. A change became apparent generally in 1985 and this appears to have been sustained in 1986–87. Nevertheless, a substantial proportion of homosexual men studied continue to practice high risk sexual practices, such as anal intercourse, including relationships with casual partners.

1. INTRODUCTION

(a) General

Because of the long incubation period from HIV infection to AIDS, predictions of future cases of AIDS are determined by past and current incidence of HIV infection. Incidence of infection in an entirely susceptible population with sufficiently high rates of partner change will initially be high, but will tend to slow as the pool of susceptibles is exhausted. However, incidence may also be reduced by changes in behaviour among both infected and susceptible individuals. Change in sexual behaviour occurring at an early stage of the epidemic when the prevalence of infection is low, may have a more marked effect on incidence than change occurring later in the epidemic when high prevalence of infection makes the probability of exposure to an infected individual high, even with low rates of partner change.

In England and Wales, the majority of cases of AIDS and HIV infection have occurred among homosexual men. Studies of the risk factors for HIV infection among homosexual men have identified receptive anal intercourse as the sexual act that has the strongest independent risk for infection (Johnson 1988; Winkelstein *et al.* 1987*a*; Moss *et al.* 1987; Kingsley *et al.* 1987).

These studies have also shown a markedly increased risk of infection with increasing numbers of sexual partners. A common feature of studies has been the significant minority reporting large numbers of sexual partners (more than 500). The proportion in the population who have any homosexual experience, and those who are exclusively homosexual, is unknown. It is therefore impossible to draw a random sample of homosexual men for study. Virtually all studies of homosexual behaviour suffer from selection biases inherent in drawing samples from volunteers at homosexual meeting places etc., or from clinic samples. Despite these shortcomings, taken together, studies from clinic and non-clinic samples in the United States (U.S.A.) and the United Kingdom (U.K.) suggest that homosexual men have higher numbers of sexual partners than heterosexual men and women (Anderson & Johnson 1989); that homosexual men attending sexually transmitted disease (STD) clinics suffer higher rates of STDs than heterosexual clinic attenders, (Belsey & Adler 1981) and that numbers of sexual partners are closely correlated with the incidence of sexually transmitted diseases (Darrow et al. 1981). These patterns of behaviour among homosexual men appear to have preceded the AIDS epidemic by several decades (Darrow et al. 1981; Gebhard & Johnson 1979). These behavioural characteristics have largely determined the pattern of the AIDS epidemic in the U.K. and U.S.A. As the risk factors for AIDS emerged, the homosexual community mounted an impressive education campaign with three main messages for risk reduction: avoid unprotected, penetrative anal intercourse; reduce numbers of partners; and use condoms.

This paper examines the available evidence for changing sexual behaviour among homosexual men in England and Wales in response to the HIV epidemic. We have examined indirect and direct evidence from trends in rates of sexually transmitted diseases (STDs), HIV prevalence and incidence, and studies of sexual behaviour.

(b) United States of America

Evidence from eight cohort studies in the U.S.A. indicates that HIV was present in the homosexual population at least from the late 1970s. The maximum incidence of HIV infection in homosexual men (i.e. the percentage of uninfected men becoming infected) occurred in the years 1980–84 and fell from 1984 onwards (Centers for Disease Control (CDC) 1987). For example, in the only cohort study based on a random sample of homosexual men in San Francisco, annual infection rates fell from an estimated 18.4% per year from 1982–84 to 4.2% in the first half of 1986 (Winkelstein et al. 1987b). From 1983 onwards, and possibly earlier, there was evidence of changing sexual behaviour among homosexual men in the U.S.A. with reduction in partner numbers; reduction in the practice of anal intercourse; and an increase in the use of condoms (Centers for Disease Control 1987b; Johnson 1988; McCusick et al. 1985; Martin 1987; Winkelstein et al. 1987b).

There is evidence from the San Francisco Men's Health Study that the falling incidence coincided with behaviour changes (Winkelstein et al. 1987b). However, behavioural change has not always led to a fall in incidence of HIV in heavily infected groups. In a cohort of 378 homosexual men, Stevens et al. (1986) recorded an annual seroconversion rate ranging from 5.5% to 10.6% between 1979 and 1983, the highest incidence occurring in the later years despite an observed reduction in sexual activity. This reflects the increasing risk of infection from one sexual partner as the prevalence of infection in the population increases. Thus behavioural risk reduction will only reduce the incidence of infection if it is of a magnitude sufficient to outweigh increased risk inherent in the rising prevalence, or occurs at an earlier stage in the epidemic, when infection rates are low.

In the city clinic cohort in San Francisco, prevalence of infection continued to increase at a virtually linear rate between 1978 and 1984, reaching over 70 % in 1985 despite observed behaviour changes over the same time period (Centers for Disease Control 1985 a). In cohorts where prevalence was already very high at the time of behaviour change, subsequent falling incidence may partly be a result of depletion of susceptibles.

(c) England and Wales

An estimated 10 % of cases of sexually transmitted disease in men in England and Wales occur in homosexual men (Belsey & Adler 1981). Information on sexuality is not recorded in statutory returns from STD clinics so trends in incidence of STDs in homosexual men can only be derived from trends for all men or by special studies.

(i) Gonorrhoea

Rates of post-pubertal gonorrhoea in men and women in England showed a slow decline in the years 1976–84. In the years 1985–86 there was a more marked reduction in rates in men from 201 per 100000 in 1985 to 170 per 100000 in 1986 (figure 1; Chief Medical Officer 1987).

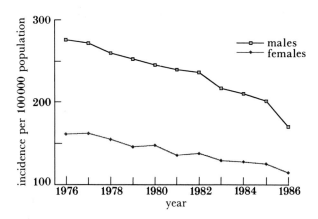

FIGURE 1. Incidence rate of post pubertal gonorrhoea per 100000 population. New cases at NHS genito-urinary medicine clinics, 1976–86. The denominator for rates is the population aged 15–59. (Source: Statistical Bulletin DHSS 2 July 1988.)

In some genito-urinary medicine clinics in London there has been a marked decline, beginning in 1981, in the proportion of homosexual male attenders with gonorrhoea; at The Middlesex Hospital the rate fell from 19 % in 1981 to only 2.3 % in 1987 (Loveday et al. 1989; Weller et al. 1984). At St Mary's Hospital male rectal gonorrhoea isolates, which occurred only in homosexual men, fell by 53 % between 1983–84 and 1986 (Gellan & Ison 1986). At the same time, the number of urethral isolates from homosexual men fell by 70 % and among heterosexual men by 30 %. In 1986 and 1987 there was a marked decline in laboratory reports of rectal gonorrhoea in males in England and Wales (PHLS Communicable Disease Surveillance Centre, unpublished data); the number of reports received annually from consistently reporting laboratories fell from an average of 505 in the years 1983–85 to 158 in 1987.

(ii) *Syphilis*

Primary and secondary syphilis in males in England is generally homosexually acquired.
Between 1976 and 1984 annual age-specific rates for new cases in males were declining slowly
(figure 2; Chief Medical Officer 1987). In 1985 and 1986 this decline was markedly
accelerated particularly in the age groups 20–24, 25–34 and 35–44 years.

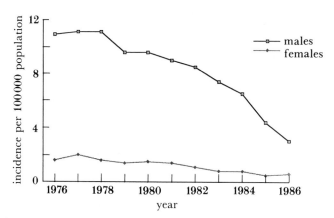

FIGURE 2. Incidence of primary and secondary syphillis per 100000 population. New cases at NHS genito-urinary
medicine clinics, England 1976–86. The denominator for rates is the population aged 15–59. (Source:
Statistical Bulletin DHSS 2 July 1988.)

(iii) *Acute hepatitis B*

Infection with hepatitis B is common among homosexual men. In many cases infection may
be acquired asymptomatically. Carne *et al.* (1987) reported a prevalence of 40–50% in
unselected homosexual STD clinic attenders tested between 1982 and 1986.

Between 1980 and 1984, 8% (520) of reported cases of acute viral hepatitis B in England,
Wales and Ireland occurred among homosexual men (Polakoff 1986). The number of
homosexually acquired cases increased annually between 1980 and 1984. Subsequently the
number of reports fell from 150 in 1984 to 51 in 1987 (Polakoff 1988; S. Polakoff, personal
communication) (figure 3). It has been suggested that this fall might be partly attributable to
the recent introduction of hepatitis B vaccination for homosexual men (Adler *et al.* 1983).
However, a survey done in 1988 showed that less than a third of STD clinics in the U.K. offer
vaccination (Loke *et al.* 1989). This suggests that vaccination has probably had little impact
on changes dating back to 1984 and that the falling incidence of acute hepatitis B infection is
more likely to be attributed to changes in sexual behaviour.

(iv) *Human Immunodeficiency Virus* (HIV)

Several studies suggest that there was a rapid rise in prevalence of HIV infection among
homosexual men, particularly in London, between 1980 and 1984 (Carne *et al.* 1987;
Mortimer *et al.* 1985; Weber *et al.* 1986). Carne *et al.* (1987) demonstrated a rise in HIV
antibody prevalence from 3.7% in 1982 to 21% in 1984 in unselected anonymously tested
homosexual men attending an STD clinic in central London. This is similar to the rise in
prevalence occurring in the San Francisco City clinic cohort in 1978 to 1980 (Jaffe *et al.* 1985).
Whereas prevalence in the San Francisco cohort continued to rise over 70% by 1985, the rapid

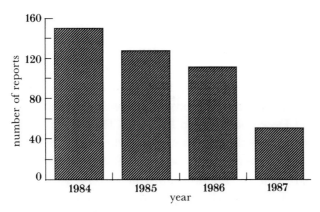

FIGURE 3. Acute hepatitis B reports in homosexual men. England and Wales 1984–1987. (Source: S. Polakoff, personal communication.)

rise in prevalence was not sustained in the London clinic study after 1984, and a prevalence of 26% was reached by the end of 1987 (Loveday *et al.* 1989). The slower rise in anti-HIV prevalence (figure 4) coincided with the continuing fall in gonorrhoea rates in the homosexual clinic population. However, figures based on serial prevalence studies must be viewed with caution because there may be underlying changes in the characteristics of the clinic population over that time (Gellan & Ison 1986).

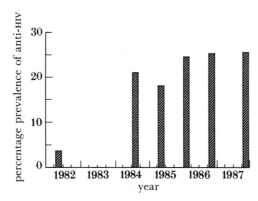

FIGURE 4. Prevalence of anti-HIV among homosexual and bisexual men attending a London genito-urinary medicine clinic 1982–87. (After Loveday *et al.* (1989).)

In a multicentre study of STD clinic attenders, mostly outside London, HIV antibody prevalence among homosexual men was relatively stable between 1985 and 1987 (around 14% in the South East and 3–6% elsewhere in the country (Collaborative Study Group 1989). These figures have been used to argue that prevalence is constant. However, the findings are difficult to interpret because of falling response rates in the clinics studied and the methodological problem of removing, from the estimate of prevalence for each year, clinic attenders who had tested positive in a previous year. Prevalence would therefore be consistently under-estimated. This problem is reflected in the work of Evans *et al.* (1989), who examined the prevalence of HIV antibody and behaviour patterns of men attending a west London clinic who requested testing for HIV antibody between 1984 and 1987. They observed a fall in antibody prevalence from 32% to 21% over the period and argue that this represents a change in behaviour. However, one alternative explanation is that as time moves on, clinics are simply testing a lower risk population. Those at highest risk have already tested positive and therefore been removed from subsequent estimates of prevalence.

There is very little data available on the incidence of HIV infection in well-defined cohorts of homosexual men. Some useful data are available from the PHLS Working Group (1989) who have obtained risk factor and HIV antibody status on 34 222 subjects tested with consent between October 1986 and December 1987 in England. The annual incidence of infection in 632 homosexual or bisexual men without HIV antibody when re-tested was 3 %. This is similar to the approximately 3 % seroconversion rate between 1985 and 1988 observed in a cohort of 240 high-risk homosexual men in London in which 6/74 (9 %) seronegative subjects subsequently seroconverted (I. V. D. Weller, personal communication). A lower incidence was observed in a cohort of 102 men in Oxford. Seven percent were initially antibody positive and over a three year period only 2 % subsequently seroconverted (Eglin et al. 1988). The increase in prevalence of 7.4 % per annum between 1982 and 1984 (Carne et al. 1987) suggests higher rates of infection at that time than the 3 % incidence subsequently observed in the studies cited above.

None of these studies can be regarded as providing a definitive statement as to the current incidence and prevalence of HIV infection in homosexual men. Taken together, they suggest that incidence may have declined since the years 1982–84, but that it has by no means ceased. A 3 % incidence rate among those already counselled and tested remains cause for concern.

(v) *Studies of sexual behaviour in homosexual men*

In a study of behaviour among homosexual men recruited through pubs, clubs and magazines in the U.K. in 1984, McManus & McEvoy (1987) documented high numbers of lifetime partners particularly among homosexual men in London, before the emergence of the AIDS epidemic.

There is now evidence that the slowing of the increase in HIV prevalence and the fall in incidence of other STDs in homosexual men occurred contemporaneously with a change in sexual behaviour. However, studies of behaviour change are often difficult to interpret, either because they are based on highly selected and heavily counselled clinic cohorts or because they are based on serial volunteer samples drawn from homosexual meeting places that may not be comparable over time.

Behaviour change among homosexual men recruited through STD clinics in London has been recorded in two cohort studies. Weber et al. (1986) showed a very marked reduction in numbers of partners per year between 1982 and 1985. Carne et al. (1987) studied behaviour change in a cohort of 100 homosexual men between 1984/5 and 1986. The median number of partners per month fell from three to one, whereas the proportion of respondents practising passive anal intercourse with more than two partners in a typical month fell from 41 to 16 %. However, only 25 % reported consistent condom use at the end of the study period.

More recently a study of homosexual men recruited from gay bars in the U.K. showed a fall in reported numbers of partners and in high risk sexual practices between 1986 and 1987, suggesting that behaviour change is currently sustained (Orton & Samuels 1988). In a study of 277 homosexual men, mostly recruited through homosexual organizations from October 1987 to July 1988, over 50 % reported condom use for anal intercourse, a higher proportion than earlier studies (R. Fitzpatrick, M. Boulton & G. J. Hart, personal communication).

Evans *et al.* (1989) documented change in the pattern of sexual behaviour among those presenting at a London STD clinic for HIV antibody testing between 1984 and 1987. This was characterized by a reduction in the proportion practising ano-receptive intercourse and in the proportion with casual partners. Nevertheless, in 1987 half of those interviewed still had casual partners. The data is difficult to interpret because of the possibly changing characteristics of those requesting antibody testing.

Data from a national (England and Wales), non-clinic based, 3 year prospective study (1985–88) of homosexual and bisexual men (project SIGMA) broadly support these trends. In London and outside, various indicators of change in sexual and related behaviour show that such change has, by and large, been consistent (McManus *et al.* 1988; Coxon & Davies 1989; Coxon 1988), involving reduction in the number of sexual (and especially in penetrative sexual) partners, changes away from receptive and insertive anal intercourse and increased use of condoms. Over the period 1985–88 the study observed a reduction of lifetime sexual partners from a median of 70 (outside London, 38) to 6 (outside London, 4) in the last year. The number of penetrative sexual partners fell to a median of 1 in all sites. However, mean values of the number of sexual (and of penetrative sexual) partners are considerably higher, reflecting an 'upper tail' of those who have not greatly reduced numbers. By 1986 the amount of anal intercourse had reduced to 9.2 % of sexual activity, engaged in by 53 % of subjects, with a further reduction to 8 % in the subsequent year. Nevertheless, a considerable amount of anal intercourse continues to be unprotected, both among couples and with casual contacts. Condoms have been adopted by 78 % of those engaging in receptive anal intercourse but quite often men do not persist in their use, continue to avoid them in high-risk sexual activity, or have (more recently) given them up (McManus *et al.* 1988; McManus & Davies 1989; Coxon & Davies 1989; Coxon 1988).

2. CONCLUSION

Much of the evidence for changes in sexual behaviour among homosexual men is based on indirect measures, such as trends in incidence of other STDs rather than on direct measures of behaviour change. Because of the social, legal and ethical constraints that have constantly accompanied the public health response to the HIV epidemic, there are very few studies that have been able to measure HIV incidence and behaviour change in representative samples of homosexual men, or indeed in any other population sub-group.

Despite the methodological problems surrounding much of the evidence presented here, different direct and indirect approaches point to the same conclusion.

There has been a recent change in sexual behaviour among homosexual men in England and Wales characterized by a reduction in numbers of partners and adoption of safer sexual behaviour. In particular places this change may have begun as early as 1983. Subsequently, a marked change became generally apparent in 1985 and this was sustained in 1986 and 1987.

The magnitude of this change has been adequate to quite dramatically reduce the incidence of other STDs including acute hepatitis B. It has not, however, been adequate to eradicate new HIV infection. The finding of a 3 % seroconversion rate per year in those previously tested, though not representative of all homosexual men, remains cause for concern. The findings presented here suggest that the epidemic curve characteristic of many cohorts in the U.S.A. has been stemmed at an earlier stage in the U.K. than in the U.S.A. However, continued

[121]

surveillance of both behaviour and HIV antibody incidence and prevalence, which allows meaningful comparisons to be made over time, is essential, for an infection whose natural history and potential spread is still incompletely understood.

We are grateful to Ms Carol Shergold for the preparation of data and to Professor A. Coxon for data from project SIGMA. A.J. is financially supported by the Medical Research Council.

REFERENCES

Adler, M. W., Belsey, E. M., McCutchan, J. A. & Mindel, A. 1983 Should homosexuals be vaccinated against hepatitis B virus? Cost and benefit assessment. *Br. med. J.* **286**, 1621–1624.

Anderson, R. M. & Johnson, A. M. 1989 Rates of sexual partner change in homosexual and heterosexual populations in the United Kingdom. In *Sex and AIDS* (ed. B. Boller) Kinsey Institute Report. New York: Oxford University Press. (In the press.)

Belsey, E. M. & Adler, M. W. 1981 Study of STD clinic attenders in England and Wales 1978: 1. Patients versus cases. *Br J. Vener. Dis.* **57**, 285–289.

Carne, C. A., Weller, I. V. D., Johnson, A. M., Loveday, C., Pearce, F., Hawkins, A., Smith, A., Williams, P., Tedder, R. S. & Adler, M. W. 1987 Prevalence of antibodies to human immunodeficiency virus, gonorrhoea rates and changing sexual behaviour in homosexual men in London. *Lancet* i, 656–658.

Centers for Disease Control 1985a Update: acquired immunodeficiency syndrome in the San Francisco cohort study, 1978–1985. *Morbidity Mortality Weekly Rep.* **34**, 573–575.

Centers for Disease Control 1987a Human immunodeficiency virus infection in the United States: A review of current knowledge. *Morbidity Mortality Weekly Rep.* **36**, S–6.

Centers for Disease Control 1987b Self-reported changes in sexual behaviours among homosexual and bisexual men from the San Francisco city clinic cohort. *Morbidity Mortality Weekly Rep.* **36**, 187–189.

Chief Medical Officer 1987 On the state of public health. In *The annual report of the Chief Medical Officer of the Department of Health and Social Security*. London: HMSO.

Collaborative Study Group 1989 HIV infection in patients attending clinics for sexually transmitted diseases in England and Wales. *Br. med. J.* **298**, 415–418.

Coxon, A. P. M. 1988 The numbers game – gay lifestyles, epidemiology of AIDS and social science. In *Social aspects of AIDS* (ed. P. Aggleton & H. Homans), pp. 126–138. London: Falmer Press.

Coxon, A. P. M. & Davies, P. M. 1989 Sexual activity of gay men in the U.K. based upon data from sexual diaries. Working Paper 15, Project SIGMA.

Darrow, W. W., Barrett, D., Jay, K. & Young, A. 1981 The gay report on sexually transmitted diseases. *Am. J. publ. Hlth* **71**, 1004–1011.

Eglin, R. P., Chapel, H. M., Harrison, J., Morgan, B. L. & Trotter, S. 1988 Behavioural and immunological changes in the Oxford cohort of healthy gay men. *Abstract Th*II. Presented at the 1st international conference on the global impact of AIDS, London.

Evans, B. A., McLean, K. A., Dawson, S. G., Teece, S. A., Bond, R. A., MacRae, K. D. & Thorp, R. W. 1989 Trends in sexual behaviour and risk factors for HIV infection among homosexual men 1984–1987. *Br. med. J.* **298**, 215–218.

Gebhard, P. H. & Johnson, A. B. 1979 *The Kinsey data: marginal tabulations of the 1938–1963 interview conducted by the Institute for sex research*. Philadelphia: W. B. Saunders.

Gellan, M. C. A. & Ison, C. A. 1986 Declining incidence of gonorrhoea in London. A response to fear of AIDS. *Lancet* ii, 920.

Jaffe, H. W., Darrow, W. & Echenberg, F. F. *et al.* 1985 The acquired immunodeficiency syndrome in a cohort of homosexual men: a six year follow-up study. *Ann. intern. Med.* **103**, 210–214.

Johnson, A. M. 1988 Social and behavioural aspects of the HIV epidemic: a review. *J. R. statist. Soc.* A **151**, 99–114.

Kingsley, L. A., Detels, R. & Kaslow, R. *et al.* 1987 Risk factors for seroconversion to human immunodeficiency virus among male homosexuals. *Lancet* i, 345–348.

Loke, R. H. T., Murray-Lyon, I. M., Balachandran, T. & Evans, B. A. 1989 Screening for hepatitis B and vaccination of homosexual men. *Br. med. J.* **298**, 234.

Loveday, C., Pomeroy, L., Weller, I. V. D., Quirk, J., Hawkins, A., Smith, A., Williams, P., Tedder, R. S. & Adler, M. W. 1989 Human immunodeficiency viruses in patients attending a sexually transmitted disease clinic in London, 1982–7. *Br. med. J.* **298**, 419–427.

Martin, J. L. 1987 The impact of AIDS on gay male sexual behaviour patterns in New York City. *Am. J. publ. Hlth* **77**, 578–581.

McKusick, M., Horstman, W. & Coates, T. J. 1985 AIDS and sexual behaviour reported by gay men in San Francisco. *Am. J. publ. Hlth* **75**, 493–496.

McManus, T. J., Coxon, A. P. M. & Davies, P. M. 1988 Changes in homosexual behaviour in the United Kingdom, 1985–1988. In *Proceedings of the 4th International AIDS Conference, Stockholm*.

McManus, T. J. & Davies, P. M. 1989 Sexual activity of gay men in the U.K., based upon data from sexual diaries. *Working Paper* 15, Project SIGMA.

McManus, T. J. & McEvoy, M. 1987 Some aspects of male homosexual behaviour in the United Kingdom. *Br. J. sex. Med.* **14**, 110–120.

Mortimer, P. P., Jesson, W. J., Vandervelde, E. M. & Pereira, M. S. 1985 Prevalence of antibody to human T lymphotropic virus type III by risk group and area, United Kingdom 1978–84. *Br. med. J.* **290**, 1176–1178.

Moss, A. R., Osmond, D., Bacchetti, P., Chermann, J. C., Barre-Sinoussi, F. & Carlson, J. 1987 Risk factors for AIDS and HIV seropositivity in homosexual men. *Am J. Epidemiol.* **125**, 1035–1047.

Orton, S. & Samuels, J. 1988 What we have learned from researching AIDS. *J. Mkt Res. Soc.* **30**, 3–34.

PHLS Working Group 1989 Prevalence of HIV antibody in high and low risk groups in England. *Br. med. J.* **298**, 422–423.

Polakoff, S. 1986 Acute viral hepatitis B: laboratory reports 1980–1984. *Br. med. J.* **293**, 37–38.

Polakoff, S. 1988 Decrease in acute hepatitis B incidence continued in 1987. *Lancet* i, 540.

Stevens, C. E., Taylor, P. E. & Zang, E. A. *et al.* 1986 Human T-cell lymphotropic virus type III infection in a cohort of homosexual men in New York City. *J. Am. med. Ass.* **255**, 2167–2172.

Weber, J. N., Wadsworth, J., Rogers, L. A., Moshtael, O., Scott, K., McManus, T., Berrie, E., Jeffries, D. J., Harris, J. R. W. & Pinching, A. J. 1986 Three year prospective study of HTLV III/LAV infection in homosexual men. *Lancet* i, 1179–1182.

Weller, I. V. D., Hindley, D. J., Adler, M. W. & Meldrum, J. T. 1984 Gonorrhoea in homosexual men and media coverage of the acquired immune deficiency syndrome in London 1982–3. *Br. med. J.* **289**, 1041.

Winkelstein, W., Lyman, D. M., Padian, N., Grant, R., Samuel, M., Wiley, J. A., Anderson, R. E., Lang, W., Riggs, J. & Levy, J. A. 1987a Sexual practices and risk of infection by the human immunodeficiency virus. *J. Am. med. Ass.* **257**, 312–325.

Winkelstein, W., Samuel, M., Padian, N., Wiley, J. A., Lang, W., Anderson, R. E. & Levy, J. A. 1987b The San Francisco men's health study: III. Reduction in human immunodeficiency virus transmission among homosexual/bisexual men, 1982–1986. *Am. J. publ. Hlth* **76**, 685–689.

Phil. Trans. R. Soc. Lond. B **325**, 163–173 (1989)   [163]

Printed in Great Britain

ESTIMATING THE SIZE OF THE HIV EPIDEMIC BY USING MORTALITY DATA

By ANNA McCORMICK

PHLS Communicable Disease Surveillance Centre, 61 Colindale Avenue, London NW9 5EQ and Office of Population Censuses and Surveys, St Catherines House, 10 Kingsway, London WC2B 6JP, U.K.

Evidence that more people are dying as a result of HIV infection than is reflected by the number of deaths among reported cases meeting the WHO definition of AIDS is derived from mortality data. Ninety-five causes of death likely to be associated with HIV infection were selected. Standardized mortality ratios due to these causes increased for single men aged 15–54 years from 100 in 1984 to 118 in 1987. The age, sex, marital status, temporal and geographic distribution of these excess deaths suggest that they are HIV-associated. It is estimated that 58 % of excess deaths due to HIV-related causes were among cases reported to the CDSC AIDS Surveillance Programme in 1987. Some of these deaths may have been among HIV-positive people who did not meet the WHO definition at the time of death. There is a need for surveillance to be extended to include HIV-positive people who die before meeting the WHO definition if the full extent of the HIV epidemic is to be identified.

1. INTRODUCTION

The epidemic of human immune deficiency virus type 1 (HIV-1) infection in England and Wales is monitored by using data from sources described in this volume and elsewhere (McCormick 1987). Identification of cases depends upon voluntary reporting of positive laboratory tests for HIV and on people with acquired immune deficiency syndrome (AIDS) meeting the World Health Organisation (WHO) definition (Centres for Disease Control 1987). Additional cases are identified from death entries on which AIDS or HIV infection is certified as a cause of death. It is uncertain how many of these fulfil the WHO definition of AIDS unless the doctor signing the medical certificate of cause of death subsequently responds to an invitation to report the case to the PHLS Communicable Disease Surveillance Centre (CDSC).

Data published monthly by the Department of Health presenting the number of deaths include only those deaths known to have occurred among people meeting the WHO definition who have been reported to the CDSC AIDS surveillance programme. Universal use of the standard WHO definition allows comparison with data collected in other countries. There is evidence, however, that there may be nearly as many deaths again among people who are infected with HIV, who have developed AIDS but have not been reported to the CDSC programme, or who have died as a result of their HIV infection without developing AIDS.

Reported causes of death among people who are HIV-positive but do not fulfil the WHO definition of AIDS include bacterial pneumonia (Selwyn *et al.* 1988; Stoneburner *et al.* 1988; Wilkes *et al.* 1988), pulmonary embolus (Selwyn *et al.* 1988; Wilkes *et al.* 1988), bacteraemia (Krumholz *et al.* 1988), various cardiac conditions (Wilkes *et al.* 1988) including endocarditis (Afessa *et al.* 1988; Galli *et al.* 1988), myocarditis and pericarditis (Marche *et al.* 1988;

Anderson *et al.* 1988), myocardial infarction (Galli *et al.* 1988) and cardiomyopathy (Zasso *et al.* 1988), febrile episodes (Periman *et al.* 1988), metabolic problems (Chirgwin *et al.* 1988), cerebral haemorrhage (Selwyn *et al.* 1988), suicide (Afessa *et al.* 1988; Rajs *et al.* 1988; Marzuk *et al.* 1988) and drug overdose (Selwyn *et al.* 1988; Afessa *et al.* 1988; Galli *et al.* 1988), gastrointestinal haemorrhage (Selwyn *et al.* 1988; Afessa *et al.* 1988), peptic ulcer (Wilkes *et al.* 1988), gastroenteritis (Moreno *et al.* 1988), pancreatitis (Wilkes *et al.* 1988), acute renal tubular necrosis (Wilkes *et al.* 1988) and many cancers (Galli *et al.* 1988; Kahn *et al.* 1988; Tirelli *et al.* 1988; Holtzman *et al.* 1988). For some deaths due to these and other causes, though occurring in people with AIDS, the stated cause(s) of death on the medical certificate may not have included AIDS or HIV infection. Most studies of mortality have been carried out on cohorts of men known to have been HIV-positive. Other than in England and Wales (McCormick 1988) no studies have been published that attempt to identify trends in the general or selected groups of the population for causes other than AIDS that were likely to be associated with HIV infection.

This paper describes how mortality data for England and Wales have been used to estimate the full extent of HIV infection severe enough to cause death, and the possible short fall in the number of cases identified when the WHO definition of AIDS is used as the criterion for acceptance.

2. Evidence for more deaths due to HIV infection than reflected in reported number of deaths among cases of AIDS

2.1. *Standardized mortality ratios (SMRs)*

SMRs for all causes of death for both men and women aged 15–54 years in England and Wales have fallen from 100 in 1980 to 83.3 for men and 84.7 for women in 1987 (figure 1).

Every death entry in which AIDS or HIV is mentioned is coded ICD 279.1 (deficiency of cell-mediated immunity) unless an underlying cause of death unlikely to be associated with HIV infection is stated. To study the possible effect of HIV infection, 95 causes of death were selected because they are included in the WHO definition of AIDS, or because they have been mentioned on the certificates of persons known to have had AIDS. These causes, which include ICD 279.1, were considered to be possibly HIV-related. SMRs for these causes alone for men who never married aged 15–54 years have increased from 100 in 1984 to 109 in 1985, 113 in 1986 and 118 in 1987 (figure 2, table 1).

Comparable figures for women who never married are 99 in 1985, 103 in 1986 and 101 in 1987. For men of all marital states other than those who never married, SMRs are 100 in 1985, 102 in 1986 and 99 in 1987 (table 2). The baseline was taken as 1984 because a change at the beginning of 1984 in the method of coding underlying cause of death makes comparison with previous years by selected causes invalid. SMRs for men who never married aged 15–54 years due to the same HIV-related ICD codes indicate however that death rates fell between 1980 and 1983 (table 3). No data on marital status was recorded on death entries during 1981.

2.2. *Rates by 5-year age groups*

For men who never married aged 15–49 years, mortality rates due to HIV related causes have increased in each 5-year age group since 1984 (table 4). The increase between 1984 and 1987 was greatest in 30–34 year olds (43%) but also high for 35–39 year olds (38%) and 40–44

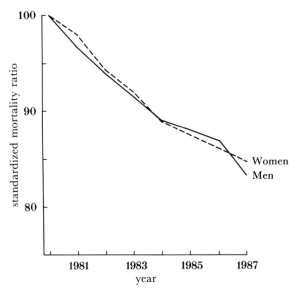

FIGURE 1. Standardized mortality ratios, all causes, all marital states, aged 15–54 years.

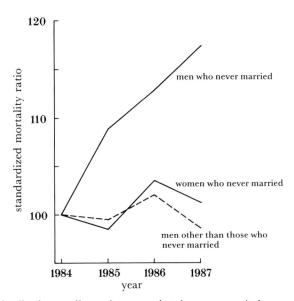

FIGURE 2. Standardized mortality ratios, HIV-related causes, marital state, aged 15–54 years.

year olds (39%). There was no similar increase among men of all marital states other than those who never married (table 4).

The age distribution at the time of death is similar to that among men with AIDS reported to CDSC who are known to have died; among these there are more deaths among 35–39 and 40–44 year olds than any other five-year age group.

2.3. Geographical distribution

The greatest increase in death rates, among men who never married aged 15–54 years, due to HIV-related causes between 1984 and 1987 was in North West Thames, North East Thames, South East Thames and North Western Regional Health Authorities (figure 3, table 5).

This is still true for HIV-related causes excluding deaths coded ICD 279.1, although in two of

ANNA McCORMICK

TABLE 1. STANDARDIZED MORTALITY RATIOS DUE TO HIV-RELATED CAUSES:
MEN WHO NEVER MARRIED AGED 15–54 YEARS, (1984–1987)

(Obs., observed; pop., population in thousands; exp., expected; 1984 = 100.)

		1984			1985	
age	obs.	pop.	exp.	obs.	pop.	exp.
15–19	282	2064.6		264	2021.5	276
20–24	370	1671.5		417	1747.2	387
25–29	232	707.1		272	769.5	252
30–34	166	329.3		211	339.5	171
35–39	146	223.0		197	231.6	152
40–44	134	143.5		157	148.7	139
45–49	175	120.3		195	121.0	176
50–54	285	119.6		275	115.6	275
total	1790	5378.9		1988	5494.6	1828
		SMR = 100			SMR = 108.8	
		1986			1987	
15–19	310	1994.6	272	309	1948.1	266
20–24	420	1794.2	397	492	1811.1	401
25–29	310	840.8	276	307	922.1	303
30–34	232	356.4	180	272	376.8	190
35–39	228	240.4	157	215	238.1	156
40–44	179	156.1	146	223	172.2	161
45–49	189	120.2	175	203	121.3	176
50–54	242	112.2	267	230	110.1	262
total	2112	5614.9	1870	2251	5699.8	1915
		SMR = 112.9			SMR = 117.54	

TABLE 2. STANDARDIZED MORTALITY RATIOS FOR 95 HIV-RELATED CAUSES FOR PERSONS
AGED 15–54 YEARS BY SEX AND MARITAL STATUS

(1985–1987; 1984 = 100.)

	1984	1985	1986	1987
men who never married	100	108.9	112.9	117.5
women who never married	100	98.5	103.5	101.2
men (other than those who never married)	100	99.5	102.0	98.6

TABLE 3. STANDARDIZED MORTALITY RATIOS DUE TO HIV-RELATED CAUSES:
MEN WHO NEVER MARRIED AGED 15–54

(1980–1983; (1980 = 100); Obs., observed; pop. population in thousands; exp., expected.)

		1980		1982			1983	
age	obs.	pop.	obs.	pop.	exp.	obs.	pop.	exp.
15–19	321	2069.6	334	2117.8	328.5	346	2108.2	327.0
20–24	338	1352.9	372	1492.0	372.8	378	1578.4	394.3
25–29	269	566.8	280	615.2	292.0	265	654.6	310.7
30–34	195	306.5	206	314.0	199.8	180	318.8	202.8
35–39	158	172.6	153	200.7	183.7	186	213.4	195.3
40–44	164	133.4	153	134.2	165.0	140	137.7	169.3
45–49	195	126.5	216	120.8	186.2	194	120.2	185.3
50–54	351	132.8	295	127.8	337.8	261	124.3	328.5
total	1991	4861.1	2009	5122.5	2065.7	1951	5255.6	2113.3
	SMR = 100			SMR = 97.3			SMR = 92.3	

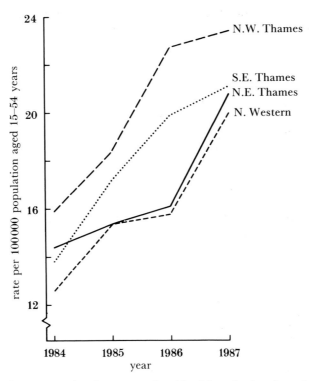

FIGURE 3. Deaths due to HIV-related causes, regional health authority of usual residence,
men who never married aged 15–54 years.

TABLE 4. DEATH RATES PER MILLION POPULATION FOR 95 HIV-RELATED CAUSES:
MEN AGED 15–54 YEARS, 1984–1987

	never married					all marital states other than never having married			
age	1984	1985	1986	1987	age	1984	1985	1986	1987
15–19	137	131	155	159	15–19	320	901	909	826
20–24	221	239	234	272	20–24	193	195	265	255
25–29	328	353	369	333	25–29	215	208	181	209
30–34	504	622	651	722	30–34	272	249	256	261
35–39	654	851	948	903	35–39	292	306	287	309
40–44	934	1056	1147	1295	40–44	424	413	429	384
45–49	1455	1612	1572	1674	45–49	592	590	616	596
50–54	2383	2379	2157	2089	50–54	878	878	921	857

the three Thames regions there was a decrease between 1986 and 1987, suggesting that for a
higher proportion of HIV-related deaths than previously, AIDS or HIV infection was stated as the
cause (figure 4). Among patients with AIDS reported to CDSC, more people who died were
reported from each of the four regions mentioned above than from any other regional health
authority (table 5).

2.4. *Temporal distribution*

The number of deaths among men of all marital states, and men who never married, aged
15–54 years, due to HIV-related causes has increased steadily each quarter year from the
beginning of 1984 to the end of 1987 (table 6). This increase is similar to that of cases reported
to CDSC by month of diagnosis (figure 5). The number of deaths among women who never

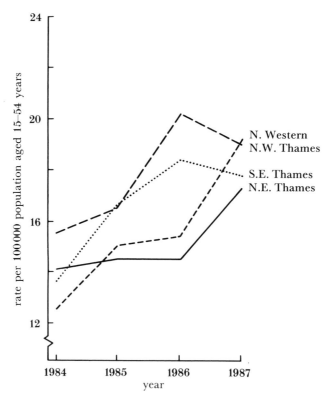

FIGURE 4. Deaths due to HIV-related causes excluding ICD 279.1, regional health authority of usual residence, never-marred men aged 15–54 years.

married also increased slightly between 1984 and 1987 but for all men except those who never married there was little change.

2.5. *Comparison of observed and expected deaths*

The number of excess deaths due to HIV-related causes in 1985, 1986 and 1987 compared with 1984 was obtained by adjusting for population changes such that

$$\text{excess deaths} = (\text{observed deaths}_i - \text{observed deaths}_0) \times \text{population}_i/\text{population}_0,$$

where $0 = 1984$ and $i = 1985$, 1986, or 1987.

Compared with 1984, among men who never married aged 15–54 years, there was an estimated excess of 159 deaths in 1985, 243 in 1986 and 354 in 1987 (table 7). There was no similar excess among men of marital states, other than those who never married, between 1985 and 1987. Among women who never married there was an estimated deficit of 11 in 1985, and an excess of 19 in 1986 and 11 in 1987, compared with 1984.

2.6. *Patients reported to CDSC who did not fulfil the WHO definition at the time of death*

Doctors are asked to report to CDSC only those patients who meet the WHO definition of AIDS. Nevertheless, by the end of June 1988, 28 patients who had died as a result of HIV infection had been reported to CDSC but have not been included in the surveillance scheme because they did not meet the WHO definition. This may be the tip of the iceberg because doctors would not be expected to report cases that they did not believe fulfilled the definition.

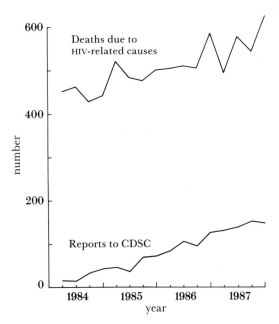

FIGURE 5. Deaths due to HIV-related causes, quarter year of registration, men who never married aged 15–54 years. Reports of AIDS cases to CDSC, quarter year of diagnosis.

TABLE 5. DEATH RATES PER 100000 POPULATION DUE TO 95 HIV-RELATED CAUSES BY REGIONAL HEALTH AUTHORITY (RHA) OF USUAL RESIDENCE, NEVER-MARRIED MEN. DEATHS AMONG CASES OF AIDS REPORTED TO CDSC BY REGIONAL HEALTH AUTHORITY OF REPORTER, ALL AGES, MEN AND WOMEN

| RHA | HIV-related causes | | | | deaths by end 1987 among cases reported to CDSC |
	1984	1985	1986	1987	
Northern	10.3	13.7	14.4	13.9	22
Yorkshire	13.4	16.1	13.5	14.1	13
Trent	11.6	12.1	11.0	11.6	8
East Anglia	9.1	11.5	12.8	12.9	12
N.W. Thames	15.9	18.4	22.7	23.4	275
N.E. Thames	14.4	15.4	16.1	20.8	137
S.E. Thames	13.8	17.2	19.9	21.1	66
S.W. Thames	17.7	16.1	15.8	17.2	27
Wessex	10.9	12.2	11.7	13.4	13
Oxford	11.5	12.3	11.4	9.8	12
South Western	12.2	13.1	13.3	13.1	18
West Midlands	11.7	11.8	14.5	12.9	15
Mersey	14.5	14.8	18.5	15.4	12
North Western	12.6	15.4	15.8	20.0	29
Wales	12.7	12.8	13.7	15.3	14

2.7. *Medical certificates stating AIDS as cause of death for persons not reported to CDSC*

Doctors who mention AIDS or HIV on the medical certificate of cause of death for a person who has not been reported to CDSC are invited to report him or her. However, despite this active follow-up in 1985 to 1987, 31 death entries mentioning AIDS or HIV for people never reported to CDSC also mentioned lymphoma, Kaposi's sarcoma, encephalopathy or an opportunistic infection, suggesting that the case would meet the WHO definition. For a further 67

TABLE 6. DEATHS DUE TO 95 HIV-RELATED CAUSES BY QUARTER YEAR OF REGISTRATION

(Persons aged 15–54 years by sex, 1984–1987.)

men who never married

	1984	1985	1986	1987
1	453	522	506	496
2	464	485	512	580
3	430	478	507	547
4	443	503	587	628
total	1790	1988	2112	2251

women who never married

	1984	1985	1986	1987
1	158	166	159	160
2	148	132	159	157
3	120	131	161	164
4	158	159	155	154
total	584	588	634	635

men (except those who never married)

	1984	1985	1986	1987
1	914	902	913	926
2	859	902	894	924
3	880	866	849	784
4	903	864	957	893
total	3556	3534	3613	3527

TABLE 7. OBSERVED AND EXPECTED EXCESS DEATHS DUE TO 95 HIV-RELATED CAUSES FOR PERSONS AGED 15–54 YEARS BY SEX AND MARITAL STATUS 1985–1987 COMPARED WITH 1984

(observed, o; expected, E)

never married men

	population (thousands)	observed, o	expected, E	excess, o–E
1984	5378.9	1790	—	—
1985	5494.6	1988	1829	159
1986	5614.9	2112	1869	243
1987	5699.8	2251	1897	354
			total	756

all men except never-married

1984	8280.7	3556	—	—
1985	8273.7	3534	3553	−19
1986	8252.5	3613	3544	69
1987	8253.1	3527	3544	−17
			total	33

never-married women

1984	4105.8	584	—	—
1985	4209.8	588	599	−11
1986	4325.1	634	615	19
1987	4390.4	635	624	11
			total	19

unreported cases, AIDS or HIV was mentioned on the death entry, either alone or with some other condition that is not included in the current WHO definition.

3. ESTIMATION OF COMPLETENESS OF REPORTING

Comparison between the number of deaths identified from death entries and deaths among cases reported to CDSC is more likely to be accurate for men who never married than for all men. Men who never married form the largest group of AIDS cases. They are a minority among men in the population aged 15–54 years and trends are therefore less biased for this group by deaths due to the 95 selected causes that are unrelated to HIV infection.

Between 1985 and 1987, there was an excess of deaths among men who never married aged 15–54 years of 756 compared with 1984. Over the same period there was an excess of deaths to men reported to be single or for whom the marital status was not known aged 15–54 years of 408 among patients with AIDS reported to CDSC compared with 1984. This suggests that only 54% of deaths due to HIV-related causes were among people with AIDS meeting the WHO definition reported to CDSC (table 8). However, during 1987 alone the proportion of cases reported to CDSC was 58%. The figure of 65% for all marital states between 1985 and 1987 compares favourably with the results of an earlier study (McCormick 1988) that suggested that only 42% of men dying from HIV infection were reported to CDSC. The improvement in reporting is largely due to active follow-up of death entries on which AIDS or HIV is mentioned, for patients not reported to CDSC at the time of death. Although this started in May 1987, retrospective follow-up increased the number of cases reported who had died in previous years.

TABLE 8. EXCESS DEATHS AS A PERCENTAGE OF EXCESS DEATHS REPORTED TO CDSC FOR MEN AGED 15–54 YEARS BY MARITAL STATUS 1985–1987 COMPARED WITH 1984

(Among cases reported to CDSC, (a); from 95 HIV-related causes on death entries, (b).)

| | all marital states | | | never-married | | |
	(a)	(b)	% reported	(a)	(b)	% reported
1985	55	136	40.4	53	159	33.3
1986	179	298	60.1	150	243	61.7
1987	253	317	79.8	205	354	57.9
total	487	751	64.8	408	756	54.0

4. CONCLUSION

There is evidence from abroad and in England and Wales that deaths have occurred due to HIV infection to persons who have not developed AIDS meeting the WHO definition. This is apparent from reports from clinicians and pathologists, and from mortality data. The temporal, geographic, age, sex and marital status distribution of increasing mortality rates due to possible HIV-related causes of death is similar to that among cases of AIDS reported to CDSC, and suggests that the trend is associated with HIV infection. The trend in mortality data derived from death certification is more marked than in deaths among people with AIDS reported to CDSC.

It is possible that only 54% of the excess deaths due to HIV-related causes in 1985–1987 identified from death certification are among cases reported to CDSC who are known to have died. This is likely to be an underestimate because it has been assumed that the 1984 baseline would remain the same in subsequent years. However, between 1980 and 1983 the standardized mortality rate for HIV-related causes fell from 100 to 92 for men who never married aged 15–54 years. It could be expected that the downward trend in deaths due to HIV-related causes but unrelated to HIV infection would have continued beyond 1983. The difference therefore between the observed and expected number of deaths in 1984–1987 is almost certainly greater than that estimated. Forward extrapolation of SMRs beyond 1983 by using 1980 as the baseline is not possible owing to the change in coding policy that resulted in approximately 11 % of deaths that would have been coded to HIV-related causes before 1984, being assigned to codes other than HIV-related causes after the beginning of 1984.

The shortfall in the number of cases reported to CDSC may be (a) because not all diagnosed AIDS cases have been reported to CDSC, (b) AIDS cases have died without being diagnosed, or (c) HIV-positive persons have died before developing AIDS. If the size of the predicted epidemic is based only on the number of cases of AIDS reported to CDSC, the result may be an appreciable underestimate of the true picture.

REFERENCES

Afessa, B., Delapenha, R., Greaves, W., Barnes, S., Saxinger, C. & Frederick, W. 1988 Clinical and epidemiologic differences between deceased AIDS and non-AIDS HIV seropositive patients (abstract). In *Proceedings of the 4th International AIDS Conference, Stockholm*, vol. 2, p. 203.

Anderson, D., Vinatea, M., Macher, A., Lopez, E., Lasala, G. & Virmani, R. 1988 Myocarditis at necropsy in patients with AIDS from mainland United States and Puerto Rico (abstract). In *Proceedings of the 4th International AIDS Conference, Stockholm*, vol. 1, p. 403.

Centres for Disease Control 1987 Revision of the CDC case definition for acquired immunodeficiency syndrome. *Morbidity Mortality weekly Rep.* **36** (suppl.), 1S.

Chirgwin, K., Rao, T. K. & Landesman, S. H. 1988 High HIV seroprevalence in patients with chronic renal failure (abstract). In *Proceedings of the 4th International AIDS Conference, Stockholm*, vol. 1, p. 402.

Galli, M., Carito, M., Cruccu, V., Zampini, L., Ciacci, D., Villa, A., Pacini, S., Zaini, G., Corsi, L., Codini, G., Saracco, A. & Lazzarin, A. 1988 Causes of death in I.V. drug abusers: a retrospective survey on 4883 subjects (abstract). In *Proceedings of the 4th International AIDS Conference, Stockholm*, vol. 2, p. 191.

Holtzman, D., Trapido, E. J., Mackinnon, J. A., Freeman, L. W., Harris, C. C., Sims, J. & Witte, J. J. 1988 AIDS and cancer: findings from a statewide registry match (abstract). In *Proceedings of the 4th International AIDS Conference, Stockholm*, vol. 2, p. 216.

Kahn, J., Desmond, S., Bottles, K., Kaplan, L., Abrams, D. & Volberding, P. 1988 Incidence of malignancies in men at San Francisco general hospital during the HIV epidemic (abstract). In *Proceedings of the 4th International AIDS Conference, Stockholm*, vol. 2, p. 328.

Krumholz, H. M., Lo, B., Hadley, K. & Sande, M. A. 1988 Community-acquired bacteraemia in AIDS patients; presentation and outcome (abstract). In *Proceedings of the 4th International AIDS Conference, Stockholm*, vol. 1, p. 399.

Marche, C., Trophilme, D., Mayorga, R., Lafont, A., Vilde, J. J. & Matheron, S. 1988 Cardiac envolvement in AIDS. A pathological study (abstract). In *Proceedings of the 4th International AIDS Conference, Stockholm*, vol. 1, p. 403.

Marzuk, P. M., Tierney, H., Tardiff, K., Gross, E. M., Morgan, E. B., Hsu, M.-A. & Mann, J. J. 1988 Increased risk of suicide in persons with AIDS. *J. Am. med. Ass.* **259**, 1333–1337.

McCormick, A. 1988 Trends in morbidity statistics in England and Wales with particular reference to AIDS from 1984 to April 1987. *Br. med. J.* **296**, 1289–1292.

McCormick, A., Tillett, H., Bannister, B. & Emslie, J. 1987 Surveillance of AIDS in the United Kingdom. *Br. med. J.* **295**, 1466–1469.

Moreno, A., Mallolas, J., Latorre, X., Gatell, J. M., Miro, J. M., Mensa, J., Valls, M. E., Gonzalez, J., Ribalta, T. & Soriano, E. 1988 Infectious gastroenteritis in AIDS patients (abstract). In *Proceedings of the 4th International AIDS Conference, Stockholm*, vol. 1, p. 404.

Periman, D. C., Fenn, M., Nyquist, P. & Harris, C. 1988 Hospitalized febrile episodes in HIV-1 infected largely intravenous drug using patients (abstract). In *Proceedings of the 4th International AIDS Conference, Stockholm*, vol. 1, p. 400.

Rajs, J., Karlsson, T. & Eklund, B. 1988 HIV-related deaths outside hospital in Stockholm (abstract). In *Proceedings of the 4th International AIDS Conference, Stockholm*, vol. 2, p. 207.

Selwyn, P. A., Schoenbaum, E. E., Hartel, D., Klein, R. S., Davenny, K. & Friedland, G. 1988 AIDS and HIV-related mortality in intravenous drug abusers (abstract). In *Proceedings of the 4th International AIDS Conference, Stockholm*, vol. 2, p. 193.

Stoneburner, R., Laussucq, S., Benezra, D., Sotheran, J. & Des Jarlais, D. 1988 Increasing pneumonia mortality in NYC, 1980–1986: Evidence for a larger spectrum of HIV-related disease in intravenous drug abusers (abstract). In *Proceedings of the 4th International AIDS Conference, Stockholm*, vol. 1, p. 411.

Tirelli, U., Tourani, J. M., Vaccher, E., Foa, R., Raphael, M., Toladano, M., Pedersen, C., Rezza, G., Monfardini, S. & Andrieu, J. M. 1988 A report of 53 patients with HIV-associated Hodgkin's disease in Europe (abstract). In *Proceedings of the 4th International AIDS Conference, Stockholm*, vol. 2, p. 327.

Wilkes, M. S., Fortin, A., Felix, J., Godwin, T. & Thompson, W. 1988 The utility of the autopsy in acquired immunodeficiency syndrome (abstract). In *Proceedings of the 4th International AIDS Conference, Stockholm*, vol. 2, p. 307.

Zasso, J.-F., Lafont, A., Chappuis, P., Chalas, J., Sayegh, F., Darwiche, H. & Camus, F. 1988 Non obstructive cardiomyopathy and selenium deficiency in AIDS (abstract). In *Proceedings of the 4th International AIDS Conference, Stockholm*, vol. 1, p. 400.

Phil. Trans. R. Soc. Lond. B **325**, 175–178 (1989)   [175]

Printed in Great Britain

RATE OF GROWTH OF AIDS EPIDEMIC IN EUROPE: A COMPARATIVE ANALYSIS

BY A. MARIOTTO†

Department of Mathematics, Imperial College of Science and Technology, London SW7 2BZ, U.K.

Estimates of the rate of increase of the AIDS epidemic for each of 18 European countries are obtained by fitting a Poisson process with exponential rate of growth to data. A linear regression model of these estimates on the proportion of cases that are intravenous drug users, homosexuals/bisexuals and heterosexuals, was estimated and suggested that the rates of growth of the epidemics amongst these groups are different and in increasing order. Empirical Bayes estimates of the rates are obtained for each country.

1. INTRODUCTION

The work in this paper has a two-fold aim. One is to compare the incidence of AIDS in the different European countries and the other is to explore the use of empirical Bayes methods for improving prediction of the growth of the epidemic, especially for the U.K. The key idea of the latter is that under certain plausible assumptions the best estimate of a parameter describing the U.K. experience, for example, is a weighted combination of the estimate from the U.K. data, and of that from other countries where the situation is similar. The gain from using the empirical Bayes approach is small so the main emphasis of the paper is on the former aim.

The data are summarized in table 1, showing the numbers of AIDS cases reported quarterly in 1986 and 1987, and total numbers reported before 1986. They are taken from a report of the World Health Organization (WHO) collaborating centre on AIDS. Countries reporting very few cases have been omitted. These include Bulgaria, East Germany, Hungary, Iceland, Luxemburg, Malta, Poland, Romania and the U.S.S.R.

One possibility is to analyse the total numbers of cases per million of population. This shows enormous variation between countries. It is likely, however, that the growth rate of the epidemic, as measured by an effective doubling time, is much more stable; therefore, we have concentrated on the analysis of the growth rate.

2. INITIAL ANALYSIS

Whereas there is strong evidence, especially for the U.K., of a slowing down from exponential growth for the spread of AIDS, it is reasonable to postulate a Poisson process of exponentially increasing rate in order to model the results presented in table 1; i.e. to suppose for each country that the rate of occurrence of cases at time t is

$$\alpha\, e^{\beta t},$$

where α and β are different for each country. In view of the remarks above we concentrate on the study of β. The emphasis is not on extrapolation but rather on summarizing the data.

† Present address: IAC-CNR, Viale del Policlinico, 137, Rome 00161, Italy.

TABLE 1. TOTAL NUMBER OF AIDS CASES REPORTED IN 18 EUROPEAN COUNTRIES

country	Mar. 1986	Jun. 1986	Sep. 1986	Dec. 1986	Mar. 1987	Jun. 1987	Sep. 1987	Dec. 1987
Austria	34	36	44	54	72	93	120	139
Belgium	160	171	180	207	230	255	277	277
Denmark	80	93	107	131	150	176	202	228
Finland	11	11	14	14	19	19	22	24
France	707	859	1050	1221	1632	1980	2532	3073
F.R.G.	459	538	675	826	999	1133	1400	1669
Greece	14	22	25	35	42	49	78	88
Ireland	8	9	10	12	14	19	19	25
Israel	23	24	31	34	38	39	43	47
Italy	219	300	367	523	664	870	1104	1411
Netherlands	120	146	180	218	260	308	370	420
Norway	21	24	26	35	45	49	64	70
Portugal	24	28	40	46	54	67	81	90
Spain	145	177	201	264	357	508	624	789
Sweden	50	57	76	90	105	129	143	163
Switzerland	113	138	170	192	227	266	299	355
U.K.	287	340	512	610	729	870	1067	1227
Yugoslavia	3	3	3	8	10	11	21	26

The model specifies that for a particular country the numbers of AIDS cases, N_j, in (t_{j-1}, t_j) $(j = 0, ..., s)$, with $t_{-1} = -\infty$, follow Poisson distributions with means

$$\int_{-\infty}^{t_0} \alpha \exp(\beta t) \, dt = \alpha \exp(\beta t_0)/\beta = \alpha \omega_0(\beta),$$

$$\int_{t_{j-1}}^{t_j} \alpha \exp(\beta t) \, dt = \alpha \exp(\beta t_j) (1 - e^{-\beta d_j})/\beta = \alpha \omega_j(\beta),$$

for $j = 1, ..., s$, where $d_j = t_j - t_{j-1}$.

TABLE 2. ESTIMATED EXPONENTIAL RATES OF INCREASE FOR 18 EUROPEAN COUNTRIES

(Based on report of the WHO Collaborating Centre on AIDS. Doubling time is $0.693/\beta$ yr. est., estimated; emp., empirical; IDU., intravenous drug users; HE., heterosexuals; HOM., homosexuals/bisexuals; s.e., standard error.)

	est. $\hat{\beta}$ (per year)		fitted $\hat{\beta}^*$ from (3) (per year)		emp. Bayes (per year)		% IDU	% HE.	% HOM.
	(a) est.	(b) s.e.	(c) est.	(d) s.e.	(e) est.	(f) s.e.	(g)	(h)	(i)
Austria	0.834	0.081	0.807	0.041	0.823	0.062	23	2	5
Belgium	0.304	0.028	0.416	0.111	0.313	0.027	2	58	25
Denmark	0.585	0.048	0.661	0.046	0.601	0.043	2	5	84
Finland	0.447	0.124	0.618	0.041	0.553	0.076	4	17	71
France	0.851	0.017	0.724	0.038	0.847	0.017	12	5	62
F.R.G.	0.731	0.021	0.714	0.042	0.731	0.021	9	3	75
Greece	0.985	0.116	0.571	0.848	0.741	0.074	1	23	47
Ireland	0.803	0.161	0.846	0.045	0.834	0.083	30	3	27
Israel	0.394	0.081	0.684	0.052	0.514	0.062	2	0	61
Italy	1.033	0.030	1.054	0.094	1.035	0.029	64	4	21
Netherlands	0.687	0.040	0.687	0.048	0.687	0.037	4	2	87
Norway	0.681	0.098	0.677	0.041	0.679	0.069	6	7	79
Portugal	0.710	0.089	0.547	0.064	0.636	0.066	6	35	51
Spain	0.997	0.039	0.999	0.076	0.997	0.036	53	1	25
Sweden	0.641	0.061	0.639	0.047	0.641	0.052	0	7	81
Switzerland	0.636	0.041	0.744	0.035	0.652	0.038	19	10	63
U.K.	0.717	0.024	0.665	0.047	0.714	0.024	2	4	85
Yugoslavia	1.317	0.273	0.810	0.042	0.867	0.091	28	8	40

Maximum likelihood estimates of α and β are the solutions of

$$\hat{\alpha} = \sum n_j / \sum \omega_j(\hat{\beta}), \tag{1}$$

$$\sum n_j \omega_j'(\hat{\beta}) / \omega_j(\hat{\beta}) = (\sum n_j) [\sum \omega_j'(\hat{\beta})] [\sum \omega_j(\hat{\beta})]^{-1}. \tag{2}$$

Note that (2) is independent of the overall incidence rate $\hat{\alpha}$. This is related to the fact that, conditional on the total number of cases $\sum N_j$, $(N_0, ..., N_s)$ have a multinomial distribution with probabilities $\omega_j(\beta) / \sum \omega_k(\beta)$, not involving α. The maximum likelihood estimate of β from the conditional distribution satisfies (2).

The variances, $\hat{v}_\beta$ of the resulting estimates can be calculated via standard methods.

Table 2 (columns (a) and (b)) shows the estimates of $\hat{\beta}$ and their standard errors. Note that $\hat{\beta}$ is in yr^{-1} and that the population doubling time is $0.69/\beta$ yr.

3. FURTHER ANALYSIS

Most of the estimates in table 2 lie between 0.6 and 1 and although considering the nature of the data, this is not a very wide range, the differences are highly significant statistically and large enough to be of genuine importance. It is therefore necessary to try to explain as much of the variation as possible in systematic terms. The only basis we have for this lies in the proportions of cases of various types, as summarized in the right-hand section of table 2.

Note that:

(i) Belgium has a very low rate of increase in the number of AIDS cases. It also has a high proportion (58%) of heterosexual cases and known special circumstances. This is however some indication that a heterosexual (HE) epidemic would grow more slowly than one driven from the other sources.

(ii) The Mediterranean countries except for Israel have high values of β and also high proportions of intravenous drug users (IDUs).

Maximum likelihood estimates of the fitting of a normal model with mean

$$\beta = \theta_0 + \theta_1(\% \text{ IDU}) + \theta_2(\% \text{ HE}), \tag{3}$$

and variance

$$\tau^2 + \hat{v}_\beta.$$

gave

parameter	estimate (per year)	s.e. (per year)
θ_0	67.14	5.47
θ_1	0.62	0.19
θ_2	−0.46	0.23

and estimate of τ as 0.097 (yr^{-1}). The fitted rates of increase for each country and corresponding standard errors are displayed in table 2 (columns (c) and (d)).

The estimated model suggests, but of course does not prove, that the rates of growth of the epidemics amongst heterosexual, homosexual/bisexual and IDUs are different and in increasing order. A direct check of this hypothesis has not been attempted here.

Clearly, Belgium has a major effect on the inclusion of the proportion of heterosexuals in (3). The fitting of the model with Belgium deleted from the data gives

$$100\hat{\beta}^* = 64.80 + 0.64 \ (\% \text{ IDU}),$$

where the coefficient 0.64 has standard error 0.15.

Note that omission of percentage of heterosexuals (% HE) has had little effect on the coefficient of percentage of intravenous drug users (% IDU) providing some reinforcement of the suggestion that an epidemic among IDUs would have a shorter doubling time than one among homosexuals.

4. EMPIRICAL BAYES ESTIMATION

To improve the estimate of the rate of increase for a particular country, by combining the information from all the countries, we may calculate the empirical Bayes estimate of β_i and its standard error. This essentially combines the direct estimate for the country with information from the remaining countries. For the latter we use the regression estimate from the previous section. The relative weights to be attached to the two sources of information depend on the relative magnitudes of the variance of the individual estimate and of the scatter about the regression.

In fact, the Empirical Bayes estimate of β_i, $\beta_i^{EB} = \lambda_i \hat{\beta}_i + (1 - \lambda_i) \hat{\beta}_i^*$ with standard error $(\lambda_i \hat{v}_{\beta_i})^{\frac{1}{2}}$ where $\lambda_i = \tau^2 / (\tau^2 + \hat{v}_{\beta_i})$. This provides a compromise between the individual estimate $\hat{\beta}_i$ and the estimate $\hat{\beta}_i^*$ from the fitting of the 'regression' (3).

Note that the estimate directly from the U.K. is not very different from the regression estimate. Thus even if the real precision of the U.K. estimate is much lower than it purports to be there would be little gain for the U.K. from the use of empirical Bayes ideas. For some other countries, especially those for which the amount of 'local' information is small, the use of empirical Bayes methods does induce an appreciable change in the estimated parameters.

Phil. Trans. R. Soc. Lond. B **325**, 179–183 (1989)   [179]

Printed in Great Britain

SEROPOSITIVITY FOR HIV IN U.K.
HAEMOPHILIACS

AIDS GROUP OF THE UNITED KINGDOM HAEMOPHILIA CENTRE DIRECTORS
WITH THE COOPERATION OF THE U.K. HAEMOPHILIA CENTRE DIRECTORS†

The results of a third seroprevalence survey of antibody to HIV in U.K. haemophiliacs, done in 1987, are presented. Out of 3028 men with haemophilia A living in the U.K. during the period 1980–1987 who had been tested for HIV antibody, 39% were positive, and out of 517 men tested with haemophilia B, 5% were positive. For both haemophilia types the proportion of seropositive men is greater among patients with a severe coagulation defect. No new seroconversions are known to have taken place after November 1986.

1. INTRODUCTION

Two surveys of the prevalence of antibody to HIV in U.K. haemophiliacs, carried out in 1985 and 1986, have been published (AIDS Group of the United Kingdom Haemophilia Centre Directors 1986, 1988). This paper gives results of a third seroprevalence survey, done in 1987. In addition to updating the information from earlier reports, the 1987 survey collected extra information about the date of the last seronegative test in patients for whom there was a subsequent seropositive test, thus enabling a more detailed investigation of the likely dates of the more recent seroconversions than was possible previously. The information from the 1987 survey, together with data from other surveys, has also enabled the cumulative incidence of AIDS in this group to be estimated. It was found that the rate of progression to AIDS was strongly dependent on age. The cumulative incidence amongst those aged less than 25 at their first seropositive test was 4% after 5 years, whereas for age groups 25–44 and 45+, 6% and 19% of patients respectively had developed AIDS. There was little evidence that the type or severity of haemophilia or the type of Factor VIII or IX that had caused HIV infection affected the rate of progression to AIDS. Details are published elsewhere (Darby *et al.* 1989).

2. PATIENTS AND METHODS

As in previous seroprevalence surveys, each of the 109 haemophilia centres in the U.K. was sent a computer printout showing the name, date of birth, and the National Haemophilia Registry number of patients with haemophilia A, B, or von Willebrand's disease who were known to have attended the centre during the period 1980–1987. The centres were asked to indicate on the printout those patients who had been tested for HIV antibody, the most recent test result and the date of the test. If the test was positive, the haemophilia centres were invited

† Report prepared by S. C. Darby, R. Doll, F.R.S., (Imperial Cancer Research Fund Cancer Epidemiology and Clinical Trials Unit, University of Oxford, Gibson Laboratories, Radcliffe Infirmary, Oxford OX2 5HE, U.K.), C. R. Rizza and R. J. D. Spooner (Oxford Haemophilia Centre, Churchill Hospital, Headington, Oxford OX3 7LJ, U.K.).

to supply the date of the first positive test and the date of the last negative test, if known. Information was requested for patients known to have died during this period as well as for those who were still alive. After the data from the 1987 survey was collated, a search was made of the results of the earlier surveys for any seropositive patients who were not included in the 1987 survey; information on these patients has been included in the present report.

All information received by August 1988 has been included, but patients known to be normally resident outside the U.K., one female patient, and one patient known to be homosexual have been excluded from the analysis.

3. RESULTS

3.1. *Prevalence of antibody to* HIV

Ninety-four of the 109 haemophilia centres in the U.K. took part in the 1987 survey and a further six centres took part only in previous surveys. Out of a total of 4401 registered haemophiliacs who received blood products in the period 1980–1987, 3545 (81 %) are known to have been tested (table 1), but among patients with a severe coagulation defect (factor VIII or IX level less than 2 % of average normal) the proportion tested was appreciably higher (1931 out of 2170 or 89 %). Altogether 1179 seropositive patients with haemophilia A and 27 patients with haemophilia B were identified. Among haemophilia A patients, 39 % of those tested were seropositive, whereas for those with a severe coagulation defect the proportion was 58 %. Among patients with haemophilia B the corresponding figures were 5 % and 9 % respectively. For five patients with haemophilia A who were reported to be seropositive in the 1987 survey, the date of their first positive test was not available. These have been included in table 1, but excluded from all further tables. The dates of earliest seropositivity ranged from December 1979 to November 1987 for haemophilia A patients and from February 1984 to September 1987 for haemophilia B patients (table 2). Explicit dates of the last negative test were available for 329 (28 %) of the seropositive patients with haemophilia A, and 12 (44 %)

TABLE 1. NUMBERS OF PATIENTS WITH HAEMOPHILIA A OR B REGISTERED IN U.K. WHO RECEIVED BLOOD PRODUCTS DURING 1980–1987, AND NUMBERS OF PATIENTS REPORTED AS TESTED AND FOUND TO BE SEROPOSITIVE IN THE THREE PREVALENCE SURVEYS, BY FACTOR VIII OR IX LEVEL

(Figures shown are totals for all three surveys. Patients known to have died since 1980 are included and patients who usually live overseas are excluded, as is one female patient and one known homosexual.)

	factor VIII or IX level (% of average normal)				
	< 2	2–10	> 10	unknown	total
haemophilia A:					
number registered	1890	1125	612	84	3711
number reported tested	1688	894	430	16	3028
number reported positive	972	164	39	4	1179
haemophilia B:					
number registered	280	279	107	24	690
number reported tested	243	209	57	8	517
number reported positive	21	5	1	0	27
all patients:					
number registered	2170	1404	719	108	4401
number reported tested	1931	1103	487	24	3545
number reported positive	993	169	40	4	1206

TABLE 2. CALENDAR DISTRIBUTION OF REPORTED DATES OF EARLIEST SEROPOSITIVE TESTS FOR PATIENTS WITH HAEMOPHILIA A OR B

(Many patients may well have seroconverted substantially before their first seropositive test.)

		haemophilia A patients	haemophilia B patients	all patients
1979	Jly–Dec.	1	—	1
1980	Jan.–Jun.	6	—	6
	July–Dec.	12	—	12
1981	Jan.–Jun.	9	—	9
	Jly–Dec.	13	—	13
1982	Jan.–Jun.	20	—	20
	Jly–Dec.	29	—	29
1983	Jan.–Jun.	26	—	26
	Jly–Dec.	56	—	56
1984	Jan.–Jun.	71	2	73
	Jly–Dec.	205	6	211
1985	Jan.–Jun.	454	9	463
	Jly–Dec.	187	5	192
1986	Jan.–Jun.	41	2	43
	Jly–Dec.	31	1	32
1987	Jan.–Jun.	9	0	9
	Jly–Dec.	4	2	6
	total	1174	27	1201

TABLE 3. CALENDAR DISTRIBUTION OF REPORTED DATES OF LAST SERONEGATIVE TEST FOR PATIENTS WITH HAEMOPHILIA A OR B FOR WHOM A SUBSEQUENT SEROPOSITIVE TEST WAS AVAILABLE

		haemophilia A patients	haemophilia B patients	all patients
1979	Jan.–Jun.	4	—	4
	Jly–Dec.	19	—	19
1980	Jan.–Jun.	27	—	27
	Jly–Dec.	33	—	33
1981	Jan.–Jun.	16	1	17
	Jly–Dec.	21	1	22
1982	Jan.–Jun.	21	—	21
	Jly–Dec.	39	1	40
1983	Jan.–Jun.	11	3	14
	Jly–Dec.	29	—	29
1984	Jan.–Jun.	25	1	26
	Jly–Dec.	29	2	31
1985	Jan.–Jun.	45	3	48
	Jly–Dec.	6	—	6
1986	Jan.–Jun.	2	—	2
	Jly–Dec.	2	—	2
	total	329	12	341

of those with haemophilia B. The calendar distribution of dates of the last seronegative test in patients for whom a subsequent seropositive test was available is given in table 3. For 10 patients, all with haemophilia A, a seronegative test was obtained on blood taken in or after July 1985, and a later test was seropositive, so that seroconversion apparently took place in or after July 1985. Details of these patients are given in table 4. Investigation revealed that 9 of the 10

TABLE 4. DETAILS OF 10 PATIENTS WITH HAEMOPHILIA A WITH LAST NEGATIVE TEST IN JULY
1985 OR LATER WHO HAD A SUBSEQUENT POSITIVE TEST

patient number	date of birth	date of last negative test	date of first positive test	factor VIII level (% of average normal)
1	10/39	11/07/85	31/07/85	0
2	12/46	—/08/85	—/08/86	0
3	09/79	24/09/85	08/11/85	0
4	01/75	—/10/85	—/03/86	0
5	01/76	—/10/85	02/05/86	2
6	08/65	—/11/85	24/10/86	0
7	03/62	07/03/86	29/09/86	0
8	12/74	07/05/86	16/06/86	5
9	05/80	28/09/86	19/11/86	0
10	05/78	03/10/86	25/10/86	0

patients were exposed to commercial material from a company whose licence was withdrawn in November 1986 because of known seroconversion after their product. Two of the 9 (patients 3 and 8) had received only this material; the remaining 7 had received it along with other commercial preparations or with National Health Service (NHS) material. One patient (number 4), who had received material from another company as well as NHS material, converted some time between October 1985 and March 1986.

4. DISCUSSION

The estimated prevalence of antibody to HIV among patients with haemophilia A or B from this survey is very similar to that found in the earlier surveys on these patients. The earlier findings of an increased prevalence among those with a severe coagulation defect and among patients with haemophilia A as compared with haemophilia B are also confirmed. The probable reason for the different prevalences between patients with haemophilia A and haemophilia B is that, until heat treatment was introduced in the U.K. fractionation centres, most factor IX (the principal material received by patients with haemophilia B) that was used in the U.K. was derived from volunteer donor plasma collected in this country. Any commercial factor IX concentrates used, that would have been based on paid donor plasma from the U.S.A. were heat treated. In an earlier survey the prevalence of anti-HIV in patients with haemophilia B was roughly the same as that in haemophilia A patients who had received only NHS factor VIII concentrates (AIDS Group of the U.K. Haemophilia Centre Directors 1986). Heat treated commercial factor VIII concentrate was introduced into the U.K. in December 1984 and over the subsequent few weeks unheated concentrates were withdrawn. With regard to the NHS concentrates, heat-treated factor VIII became available from the Scottish National Blood Transfusion Service in December 1984 and from Blood Products Laboratory (BPL) Elstree in February 1985. By July 1985 only heat-treated factor VIII was being supplied by BPL. Heat-treated factor IX concentrate became available in August–September 1985, and by early October issues of unheated factor IX from BPL were discontinued. The period between HIV exposure and seroconversion is usually less than 14 weeks (Simmonds et al. 1988) but in rare cases it may exceed 6 months (Ranki et al. 1987). Thus the one patient who apparently seroconverted after all concentrate was heat-treated but who had not received material from the company whose licence was later withdrawn may have been infected by one of the last few batches of unheated factor VIII. Individual donor testing was in place for all concentrates by November 1986, and no seroconversions are known to have taken place in or after November 1986. This accords with the results of a recent review of the safety of products used for treating haemophilia patients carried out at the U.S.A. Centers for Disease Control that concluded that cases of HIV seroconversion associated with the use of heat-treated products are now rare (Centers for Disease Control 1988).

We gratefully acknowledge the help of Mrs Irene Stratton, Mrs Valerie Weare, and Mrs Patricia Wallace in assembling the data, Sir David Cox for helpful discussions, and Mrs Cathy Harwood for typing the manuscript.

References

AIDS Group of the U.K. Haemophilia Centre Directors 1986 Prevalence of antibody to HTLV III in haemophiliacs in the United Kingdom. A survey carried out by the AIDS Group of the United Kingdom Haemophilia Centre Directors with the co-operation of the United Kingdom Haemophilia Centre Directors. *Br. med. J.* **293**, 175–176.

AIDS Group of the U.K. Haemophilia Centre Directors 1988 Prevalence of antibody to HIV in haemophiliacs in the United Kingdom: A second survey. *Clin. Lab. Haemat.* **10**, 187–191.

Centres for Disease Control 1988 Safety of therapeutic products used for haemophilia patients. *Morbidity mortality wkly. Rep.* **37**, 441–450.

Darby, S. C., Rizza, C. R., Doll, R., Spooner, R. J. D., Stratton, I. M. & Thakrar, B. 1989 Incidence of AIDS and excess of HIV associated mortality in U.K. haemophiliacs: report on behalf of the directors of haemophilia centres in the U.K. *Br. med. J.* **298**, 1064–1068.

Ranki, A., Valle, S.-L., Krohn, M., Antonen, J., Allain, J.-P., Leuther, M., Franchini, G. & Krohn, K. 1987 Long latency precedes overt sero-conversion in sexually transmitted human-immunodeficiency-virus infection. *Lancet* ii, 589–593.

Simmonds, P., Lainson, F. A., Cuthbert, R., Sted, C. M., Peutherer, J. F. & Ludlam, C. A. 1988 HIV antigen and antibody detection: variable responses to infection in the Edinburgh haemophiliac cohort. *Br. med. J.* **296**, 593–598.

Phil. Trans. R. Soc. Lond. B **325**, 185–187 (1989)   [185]

Printed in Great Britain

PREDICTION FOR SMALL SUBGROUPS

By D. R. COX, F.R.S.[1], and A. C. DAVISON[2]

[1] *Nuffield College, Oxford OX1 1NF, U.K.*
[2] *Department of Mathematics, Imperial College, London SW7 2BZ, U.K.*

Prediction limits are calculated for the number of events likely to occur in a specified time period in an exponentially growing epidemic. The basis for the prediction is the total number of events observed in the past.

1. Introduction

In predicting the number of new cases of AIDS to be diagnosed in some future period, there are essentially three sources of error. These arise respectively from:

(*a*) use of an incorrect empirical formula or model on which to base the prediction;

(*b*) errors in estimating unknown parameters in the model, e.g. errors in estimating the doubling time were exponential growth to be assumed;

(*c*) Poisson-distributed variations in observed numbers to be anticipated even if the systematic part of the variation were to be correctly specified.

For predicting some way ahead with fairly large numbers, the first type of error is likely to predominate. This is the case, for example, in predicting the number of AIDS cases in England and Wales for three or four years ahead. This is essentially because many different shapes of curve are consistent with the data on which the prediction is based. For rather short-term prediction (*a*) becomes less important and ultimately, when predicting rather small numbers a short time ahead, Poisson type errors, (*c*), will be the major source of uncertainty. This is particularly relevant if we wish to predict events within a small geographical area for a rather short time ahead.

One approach to such a prediction would be based on a careful analysis of the spatial distribution of the epidemic leading to a small area prediction formula based on local characteristics and experience. Although this could be of considerable interest, here we develop a much simpler approach in which the total number of cases diagnosed up to the current point is used as a basis for prediction.

The central idea is to assume that the broad pattern of growth is determined via a large body of data and is essentially the same throughout but that the local rate varies from place to place and can be determined only via the total number of cases observed locally.

2. Formulation

Suppose then that in the area under study, diagnoses occur in a Poisson process of rate $b\lambda e^{bt}$, where b is a known constant but λ is unknown. Thus the doubling time is $0.693/b$ years. Suppose further that in the area or subgroup in question n_0 cases have been diagnosed up to time t_0 and that it is required to predict the number n' of new cases to be diagnosed in a future time period (t', t''). The arguments apply with minor modification if the rate is $\lambda h(t)$, where $h(t)$ is any known function of time.

Define a new time scale, which we call operational time, by

$$s(t) = e^{bt}.$$

On this time scale cases occur in a Poisson process of constant rate λ and the key time points $-\infty, t_0, t', t''$ are transformed to $0, s_0 = e^{bt_0}, s' = e^{bt'}, s'' = e^{bt''}$.

The value n' to be predicted is such that the split (n_0, n') is consistent with a binomial distribution with probability of 'success'

$$(s'' - s')/(s_0 + s'' - s') = p,$$

say; this is known.

Thus the upper and lower $1 - 2\epsilon$ limits for n' are respectively the largest n^* and the smallest n_* such that

$$\epsilon \leqslant \sum_{r=n^*}^{n_0+n^*} (1-p)^{n_0+n^*-r} p^r \binom{n_0+n^*}{r},$$

$$\epsilon \leqslant \sum_{r=0}^{n_*} (1-p)^{n_0+n^*-r} p^r \binom{n_0+n_*}{r}.$$

The values of n^* and n_* can be found numerically as set out below. A simple point estimate of n' is found by writing

$$n'/(n_0 + n') = p$$

and solving for n'.

The values of n^* and n_* are most straightforwardly found for given n_0 and p by enumeration of the probabilities:

$$p^* = \sum_{r=n^*}^{n_0+n^*} p^r (1-p)^{n_0+n^*-r} \binom{n_0+n^*}{r},$$

and

$$p_* = \sum_{r=0}^{n^*} p^r (1-p)^{n_0+n''-r} \binom{n_0+n_*}{r}.$$

Direct calculation is tedious, and a large saving in computer time is obtained by noting that

$$p^* = I_p(n^*, n_0 + 1) \quad \text{and} \quad p_* = I_{1-p}(n_0, n_* + 1),$$

where

$$I_x(a, b) = \frac{1}{B(a, b)} \int_0^x t^{a-1} (1-t)^{b-1} \, dt$$

is the incomplete beta function. Press *et al.* (1986) give FORTRAN and PASCAL algorithms for numerical evaluation of $I_x(a, b)$.

For large values of n_0 a normal approximation is available. Suppose that X is a binomial random variable with index $n_0 + n$ and probability p. Then approximately,

$$\text{pr}(X \leqslant n) = \Phi \left\{ \frac{n - (n + n_0) p}{\sqrt{[(n + n_0) p(1-p)]}} \right\} = g(n),$$

say, where $\Phi(.)$ is the standard normal cumulative distribution function. The values n_* and n^* roughly satisfy the equations $g(n) = \epsilon$ and $g(n) = 1 - \epsilon$. Thus they are the solutions of

$$An^2 + Bn + C = 0,$$

[148]

where $\quad A = (1-p)^2, \quad B = p(p-1)\,(2n+z_\epsilon^2), \quad$ and $\quad C = np[np-(1-p)\,z_\epsilon^2].$

Here $\Phi(z_\epsilon) = \epsilon$, and z_ϵ is found from tables of the normal distribution.

PASCAL programs to calculate exact and approximate values of n^* and n_* are available from the second author.

3. Numerical results

Table 1 shows the 90% prediction limits obtained from the formulae of §2; three values of doubling time have been used. The main qualitative conclusion to be drawn from the results is the surprising insensitivity to the doubling time, confirming the remarks in §1.

TABLE 1. LOCAL PREDICTIONS OF NUMBERS OF EVENTS LIKELY TO ARISE IN NEXT YEAR
AND THE YEAR AFTER NEXT

(Doubling time A: 1.25 years, B: 1.75 years, C: 2.5 years.)

number of events observed so far	next year			year after next			next 2 years combined		
	A	B	C	A	B	C	A	B	C
0	(0, 3)	(0, 2)	(0, 2)	(0, 5)	(0, 3)	(0, 2)	(0, 7)	(0, 4)	(0, 3)
2	(0, 6)	(0, 4)	(0, 3)	(0, 10)	(0, 6)	(0, 4)	(0, 14)	(0, 9)	(0, 6)
4	(0, 8)	(0, 6)	(0, 4)	(1, 14)	(0, 8)	(0, 5)	(2, 20)	(1, 13)	(0, 8)
6	(1, 13)	(0, 8)	(0, 5)	(2, 17)	(1, 10)	(0, 7)	(4, 26)	(2, 16)	(1, 11)
8	(1, 13)	(1, 9)	(0, 6)	(3, 21)	(1, 13)	(0, 8)	(6, 32)	(3, 20)	(1, 13)
10	(2, 15)	(1, 10)	(0, 7)	(5, 24)	(2, 15)	(1, 9)	(9, 37)	(5, 23)	(2, 15)
15	(5, 20)	(3, 14)	(1, 10)	(10, 33)	(5, 20)	(2, 12)	(16, 50)	(9, 31)	(5, 20)
20	(7, 25)	(4, 17)	(2, 12)	(14, 41)	(7, 24)	(3, 15)	(24, 63)	(13, 39)	(7, 25)
25	(10, 29)	(6, 20)	(3, 14)	(19, 49)	(10, 29)	(5, 18)	(32, 75)	(18, 46)	(10, 29)
30	(13, 34)	(8, 23)	(4, 16)	(24, 57)	(12, 33)	(6, 21)	(40, 87)	(23, 53)	(13, 34)
40	(19, 43)	(9, 26)	(6, 20)	(35, 72)	(18, 42)	(9, 26)	(58, 110)	(33, 67)	(19, 43)
50	(25, 52)	(11, 29)	(9, 24)	(46, 67)	(24, 51)	(13, 31)	(75, 133)	(43, 81)	(25, 51)
60	(31, 60)	(18, 41)	(11, 28)	(57, 102)	(30, 59)	(16, 36)	(93, 156)	(53, 95)	(31, 60)

The simple quadratic approximation at the end of §2 gives adequate accuracy provided that the lower limit is at least 10.

As an example, in Wales up to 30 June 1988, 27 cases had been reported so that, taking a local doubling time of 1.25 years, anything between 12 and 30 new cases could be expected in the following year.

REFERENCE

Press, W. H., Flannery, B. P., Teukolsky, S. A. & Vetterling, W. T. 1986 *Numerical recipes: the art of scientific computing.* Cambridge University Press.